PHARMACOLOGY – RESEARCH, SAFETY TESTING AND REGULATION

PRESCRIPTION DRUGS

MONITORING, SAFETY, USE AND MANAGEMENT PROGRAMS

PHARMACOLOGY – RESEARCH, SAFETY TESTING AND REGULATION

Additional books and e-books in this series can be found
on Nova's website under the Series tab.

PHARMACOLOGY – RESEARCH, SAFETY TESTING AND REGULATION

PRESCRIPTION DRUGS

MONITORING, SAFETY, USE AND MANAGEMENT PROGRAMS

KAREN SUE MCKINNEY
EDITOR

New York

NOTICE TO THE READER

Library of Congress Cataloging-in-Publication Data

ISBN: 978-1-53617-288-1

Published by Nova Science Publishers, Inc. † New York

CONTENTS

Preface		**vii**
Chapter 1	Examining FDA'S Prescription Drug User Fee Program *Committee on Energy and Commerce*	**1**
Chapter 2	Prescription Drug Monitoring Programs (Updated) *Lisa N. Sacco, Amanda K. Sarata and Johnathan H. Duff*	**125**
Chapter 3	Prescription Opioids: Patient Options for Safe and Effective Disposal of Unused Opioids *United States Government Accountability Office*	**175**
Chapter 4	Prescription Drug Use in the United States, 2015–2016 *Crescent B. Martin, Craig M. Hales, Qiuping Gu and Cynthia L. Ogden*	**201**
Chapter 5	Prescription Drug Use Among Adults Aged 40–79 in the United States and Canada *Craig M. Hales, Jennifer Servais, Crescent B. Martin and Dafna Kohen*	**213**

Chapter 6 To Amend Title XVIII of the Social Security Act to Require Prescription Drug Plan Sponsors under the Medicare Program to Establish Drug Management Programs for at-Risk Beneficiaries **223**
Committee on Energy and Commerce

Index **301**

Related Nova Publications **309**

PREFACE

The Prescription Drug User Fee Act authorized the Food and Drug Administration to collect user fees from industry to support the approval of new drugs and biologics. The Prescription Drug User Fee Agreement has been a success bringing safe and effective new products to patients in a timely manner as reported in chapter 1.

Chapter 2 provides an overview of prescription drug monitoring programs (PDMPs), including their operation, enforcement mechanisms, costs, and financing. It also examines the effectiveness of PDMPs and outlines federal grants supporting PDMPs.

Finally, it discusses relevant considerations for policymakers including interstate data sharing, interoperability, protection of health information, and the possible link between the crackdown on prescription drug abuse and rise in heroin abuse. Chapter 3 examines federally recommended and other available methods patients may use to dispose of unused prescription opioids, and what is known about patients' use of these methods.

Monitoring prescription drug use patterns at the population level can inform research and clinical practice. These patterns may shift over time in response to changing health needs, updated clinical guidelines, policy changes, and other factors. Chapters 4 and 5 examine statistics pertaining to drug use monitoring.

Chapter 6 examines bill (H.R. 5675) to amend title XVIII of the Social Security Act to require prescription drug plan sponsors under the Medicare program to establish drug management programs for at-risk beneficiaries.

Chapter 1 - This is an edited, reformatted and augmented version of Hearing Before the Subcommittee on Health of the Committee on Energy and Commerce House of Representatives, One Hundred Fifteenth Congress, First Session, Serial No. 115–18, dated March 22, 2017.

Chapter 2 - In the midst of national concern over the opioid epidemic, federal and state officials are paying greater attention to the manner in which opioids are prescribed. Nearly all prescription drugs involved in overdoses are originally prescribed by a physician (rather than, for example, being stolen from pharmacies). Thus, attention has been directed toward better understanding how opioids are being prescribed and preventing the diversion of prescription drugs after the prescriptions are dispensed. Prescription drug monitoring programs (PDMPs) maintain statewide electronic databases of prescriptions dispensed for controlled substances (i.e., prescription drugs with a potential for abuse that are subject to stricter government regulation). Information collected by PDMPs may be used to educate and inform prescribers, pharmacists, and the public; identify or prevent drug abuse and diversion; facilitate the identification of prescription drug-addicted individuals and enable intervention and treatment; outline drug use and abuse trends to inform public health initiatives; or educate individuals about prescription drug use, abuse, diversion, and PDMPs themselves. As of February 2018, 50 states, the District of Columbia, and two territories (Guam and Puerto Rico) had operational PDMPs within their borders. How PDMPs are organized and operated varies among states. Each state determines which agency houses the PDMP; which controlled substances must be reported; which types of dispensers (e.g., pharmacies) are required to submit data; how often data are collected; who may access information in the PDMP database (e.g., prescribers, dispensers, or law enforcement); the circumstances under which the information may (or must) be accessed; and what enforcement mechanisms are in place for noncompliance. PDMP costs may vary widely, with startup costs that can range as high as $450,000 to over $1.5

million and annual operating costs ranging from $125,000 to nearly $1.0 million. States finance PDMPs using monies from a variety of sources including the state general fund, prescriber and pharmacy licensing fees, state controlled substance registration fees, health insurers' fees, direct-support organizations, state grants, and/or federal grants. The federal government supports state PDMPs through programs at the Departments of Justice (DOJ) and Health and Human Services (HHS). Since FY2002, DOJ has administered the Harold Rogers Prescription Drug Monitoring Program, and in FY2017, DOJ incorporated this grant program into the new Comprehensive Opioid Abuse Program. HHS programs include National All Schedules Prescription Electronic Reporting (NASPER), State Demonstration Grants for Comprehensive Opioid Abuse Response, Opioid Prevention in States grants, State Targeted Response to the Opioid Crisis Grants, and various pilots and initiatives under the Office of the National Coordinator for Health Information Technology (ONC). Of note, NASPER last received appropriations (of $2.0 million) in FY2010. State PDMPs vary with respect to whether or how information contained in the database is shared with other states. Federal policymakers have repeatedly emphasized the importance of enhancing interstate information sharing and the interoperability of state PDMPs. In 2011, the Obama Administration included efforts to increase interstate data sharing in its action plan to counter prescription drug abuse. In 2017, a presidential commission recommended, among other things, that the Trump Administration support legislation to require DOJ to fund a "data-sharing hub" and require states receiving federal grant funds to share PDMP data. The available evidence suggests that PDMPs can be effective in reducing the time required for drug diversion investigations, changing prescribing behavior, reducing "doctor shopping," and reducing prescription drug abuse. Assessments of effectiveness should also take into consideration potential unintended consequences of PDMPs, such as limiting access to medications for legitimate use or pushing drug diversion activities over the border into a neighboring state. Experts suggest that PDMP effectiveness might be improved by increasing the timeliness, completeness, consistency, and accessibility of the data. Policy issues that might come before Congress include the role of state PDMPs in federal efforts to combat prescription drug abuse, the role of the federal government in interstate data-sharing and interoperability, and the possible link between the crackdown on prescription drug abuse and the uptick in illicit opioid (e.g., heroin and illicit fentanyl) abuse. While establishment and enhancement of PDMPs enjoy relatively broad support, stakeholders express concerns about health care versus law enforcement uses of PDMP data (particularly with regard to protection of personally identifiable health information).

Chapter 3 - In 2017, an estimated 11.1 million Americans misused a prescription pain reliever, which included opioids. This misuse contributes to opioid abuse and death, which has quintupled from 1999 to 2017; about 17,000 people died from prescription opioid overdoses in 2017. Government agencies and stakeholders have attempted to address the potential for misuse and abuse by facilitating safe disposal of unused prescription opioids and other drugs. The SUPPORT for Patients and Communities Act enacted in 2018 included a provision for GAO to review patient disposal of unused opioids, among other things. This chapter examines (1) federally recommended and other available methods patients may use to dispose of unused prescription opioids, and (2) what is known about patients' use of these methods. To do this work, GAO examined peer-reviewed, academic literature on outcomes for prescription opioid disposal; reviewed federal agency documentation; interviewed federal agency officials, independent researchers, and stakeholder group representatives—such as those from the American Medical Association; and analyzed DEA data as of April 2019 on permanent drug collection sites. GAO also interviewed representatives of three companies that manufacture commercial in-home disposal products and reviewed publicly available documents about these products.

Chapter 4 - Monitoring prescription drug use patterns at the population level can inform research and clinical practice. These patterns may shift over time in response to changing health needs, updated clinical guidelines, policy changes, and other factors. The percentage of the U.S. population that used one or more prescription drugs increased from 1999–2000 through 2007–2008. This chapter describes prescription drug use by age, sex, and race and Hispanic origin in 2015–2016 and trends over the preceding decade.

Chapter 5 - Patterns of prescription drug use may reflect underlying patterns of health conditions and health care access in the population. Polypharmacy, often defined as the simultaneous use of five or more prescription drugs, is more common in an aging population where multiple coexisting chronic conditions often occur; however, safety concerns may arise. The United States and Canada share many cultural and historical ties, but with different models for health care delivery. This chapter describes the use of one or more and five or more prescription drugs among adults aged 40–79 in the United States and Canada.

In: Prescription Drugs
Editor: Karen Sue McKinney
ISBN: 978-1-53617-288-1

Chapter 1

EXAMINING FDA'S PRESCRIPTION DRUG USER FEE PROGRAM*

Committee on Energy and Commerce

Wednesday, March 22, 2017
House of Representatives, Subcommittee on Health,
Committee on Energy and Commerce,
Washington, DC.

The subcommittee met, pursuant to call, at 10:15 a.m., in room 2322 Rayburn House Office Building, Hon. Michael Burgess (chairman of the subcommittee) presiding.

Present: Representatives Burgess, Guthrie, Upton, Blackburn, Griffith, Bilirakis, Long, Bucshon, Brooks, Hudson, Carter, Green, Engel, Butterfield, Matsui, Sarbanes, Schrader, Kennedy, Cárdenas, and Eshoo.

Staff present: Adam Fromm, Director of Outreach and Coalitions; Jay Gulshen, Legislative Clerk, Health; Carly McWilliams, Professional Staff

* This is an edited, reformatted and augmented version of Hearing Before the Subcommittee on Health of the Committee on Energy and Commerce House of Representatives, One Hundred Fifteenth Congress, First Session, Serial No. 115–18, dated March 22, 2017.

Member, Health; Alex Miller, Video Production Aide and Press Assistant; Jennifer Sherman, Press Secretary; Danielle Steele, Policy Coordinator, Health; and John Stone, Senior Counsel, Health; Jeff Carroll, Minority Staff Director; Samantha Satchell, Minority Policy Analyst; Kimberlee Trzeciak, Minority Health Policy Advisor; and C. J. Young, Minority Press Secretary.

OPENING STATEMENT OF HON. MICHAEL C. BURGESS, A REPRESENTATIVE IN CONGRESS FROM THE STATE OF TEXAS

Mr. Burgess. I ask everyone to take their seats. The subcommittee will come to order, and I will recognize myself for an opening statement for 5 minutes.

Today's hearing marks the Health Subcommittee's second opportunity to consider the reauthorization of several key FDA user fee programs. The Prescription Drug User Fee Act authorized the Food and Drug Administration to collect user fees from industry to support the approval of new drugs and biologics, and is a top priority for this committee.

This was first authorized in 1992, and while there is always room for improvement, the Prescription Drug User Fee Agreement has been a success bringing safe and effective new products to patients in a timelier manner. Every 5 years since, pursuant to a process set forth in statute, Congress has reauthorized the program after reviewing the recommendations from the Food and Drug Administration, industry, patient groups, and other stakeholders.

The committee has been reviewing the Prescription Drug User Fee Agreement since December when it was transmitted to Congress and publicly posted. As I stated in our hearing on the generic and biosimilar programs earlier this month, Chairman Walden and I are committed to shepherding the user fee legislation through committee following regular order and getting it to the House floor with ample time to spare.

Reauthorization of the user fee agreements every 5 years provides an opportunity, an opportunity to examine, an opportunity to improve upon the state of discovery, development, and delivery of medical therapies in America. For instance, in 2012, the reauthorization of the user fees in the Food and Drug Administration's Safety and Innovation Act established the Breakthrough Therapy Designation. This program expedites the review and approval of promising new drugs that show early evidence of efficacy in serious, life-threatening diseases with an unmet clinical need.

Under this program, over 165 products have been granted breakthrough designation which means more treatments, which means more cures, are being prioritized for patients suffering from some of the most debilitating conditions. I am pleased that the user fee agreements considering now will continue to build upon the success of the Breakthrough Therapy program.

A unique factor in the negotiations of these user fee agreements was its overlap with the development of the 21st Century Cures Act, a bill enacted in December of last year after a multi-Congress effort led by Representative Fred Upton and Representative Diane DeGette. Over the course of the 113th and 114th Congresses, members of this subcommittee worked to uncover opportunities to strengthen and opportunities to streamline the process by which cures are discovered and then made available to patients. The resulting law touches each step of the process through which new treatments come to the bedside.

I am encouraged to see in our witness's testimony that the Prescription Drug User Fee Agreement VI will dedicate resources to complement the implementation of the many priorities, the many priorities of the 21st Century Cures bill. In particular, I like the fact that the FDA will formalize a structure to incorporate patient input and patient experience into the benefit-risk assessment of products that are actually under development. This is a good thing. Patients have the most at stake and they deserve to be heard.

I am also encouraged that the Food and Drug Administration will dedicate resources to modernize clinical trials and evidence development including the utilization of real-world evidence in investment in biomarkers. Real-world evidence has the potential to increase sufficiency and foster robust data collection and analysis. Advancing development of biomarkers has significant promise to accelerate regulatory decision making and expedite the pace of clinical trials without sacrificing standards for efficacy and safety.

Other provisions incorporated into the proposal for PDUFA VI— OK, you made me say it—PDUFA VI. I was trying to just call it the user fee agreements—reflects the top priorities of this committee in the 21st Century Cures Act. Again I want to reiterate my commitment to ensuring that this reauthorization stays on track. We all know there are a lot of competing influences this year, but this year will mark the fifth renewal by Congress, and it is widely agreed that the prescription drug user fee agreements will provide for the timely review of new drug and new biologic license applications. Again I want to underscore that is a good thing.

I thank all of our witnesses for being here, particularly Dr. Woodcock. Thank you, and welcome again back to our humble little subcommittee for one more hearing. I look forward to hearing from each of you and more about the agreement that is before us today, and I will yield back the balance of my time.

The chair now recognizes the gentleman from Texas, the ranking member of the subcommittee, Gene Green, 5 minutes for an opening statement, please.

[The statement of Mr. Burgess follows:]

Prepared Statement of Hon. Michael C. Burgess

The Subcommittee will come to order.

The Chair will recognize himself for an opening statement.

Today's hearing marks the Health Subcommittee's second opportunity to consider the reauthorization of several key FDA user fee programs. The Prescription Drug User Fee Act (PDUFA) authorized FDA to collect user fees from industry to support the approval of new drugs and biologics, and is a top priority for this Committee. It was first authorized in 1992 and, while there is always room for improvement, PDUFA has been a remarkable success, bringing safe and effective new drug products to patients in a more timely manner. Every five years since, pursuant to a process set forth in statute, Congress has reauthorized the program after reviewing recommendations from FDA, industry, patient groups, and other stakeholders.

The Committee has been reviewing the PDUFA VI agreement since December, when it was transmitted to Congress and publicly posted. As I stated at our hearing on the generic and biosimilar user fee programs earlier this month, Chairman Walden and I are committed to shepherding the user fee legislation through Committee, following regular order, and getting it to the House floor with ample time to spare.

Reauthorization of the user fee agreements every five years provides an opportunity to examine and improve upon the state of discovery, development, and delivery of medical therapies in America. For instance, the 2012 reauthorization of PDUFA in the Food and Drug Administration Safety and Innovation Act, commonly known as FDASIA, established the Breakthrough Therapy Designation. This program expedites the review and approval of promising new drugs that show early evidence of efficacy in serious, life-threatening diseases with unmet clinical need. Under this program over 165 products have been granted breakthrough designation, which means more treatments and cures are being prioritized for patients suffering from some of the most despairing conditions. I am pleased that PDUFA VI will continue to build upon the success of the breakthrough therapy program.

A unique factor in the negotiation of PDUFA VI, was its overlap with development of the 21st Century Cures Act, a bill enacted last year after a multi-year initiative led by Representative Upton and Representative DeGette. Over the course of the 113th and 114th Congresses, members of this subcommittee worked to uncover opportunities to strengthen and streamline the process by which cures are discovered and made available to patients. The resulting law touches each step of the process through which new treatments and cures come to market. I am encouraged to see in our witnesses' testimonies that PDUFA VI will dedicate resources to complement the implementation of many of the priorities in 21st Century Cures.

In particular, I am pleased to see that FDA will formalize a structure to incorporate patient input and experience into the benefit-risk assessment of products in development. Patients have the most at stake, and they deserve to be heard. I am also encouraged to see that FDA will dedicate resources to modernize clinical trials and evidence development, including the utilization of real-world evidence and investment in biomarkers. Real-world evidence has the potential to increase efficiency and foster robust data collection and analysis. Advancing development of biomarkers has incredible promise to accelerate regulatory decision-making and to expedite the pace of clinical trials without sacrificing standards for efficacy and safety.

Numerous other provisions incorporated in the proposal for PDUFA VI reflects the top priorities of this Committee in the 21st Century Cures Act, and I want to reiterate my commitment to ensuring this reauthorization stays on track. This year will mark the fifth renewal by Congress, and it is widely agreed that PDUFA VI will provide for the timely review of new drug and biologic license applications. I thank our witnesses for being here today and I look forward to hearing more from each of you about the agreement before us today.

OPENING STATEMENT OF HON. GENE GREEN, A REPRESENTATIVE IN CONGRESS FROM THE STATE OF TEXAS

Mr. Green. Thank you, Mr. Chairman. I thank all our witnesses, both Dr. Woodcock, welcome back again, and our second panel for being here this morning. Today we are examining the sixth Prescription Drug User Fee Agreement, PDUFA VI. I think it is fair to say that we all support a strong FDA that is responsive to the needs of the patient community and the innovations of scientific research and healthcare delivery.

I am pleased that Congress is moving judicially through the process of reauthorizing the user fee programs and honoring their negotiations that have led to the agreements, and PDUFA is the most mature of the user fee programs having first been enacted in 1992. Sometimes our committee seems like we are a little mature.

The law lays out a detailed process for reauthorization that requires FDA to negotiate with industry to develop recommendations and that the agency solicit public input and hold public hearings and consult with Congress and patients and consumer advocates and other relevant parties. The recommendations that are a result of this process must also be available publicly for a period for public comment, and ultimately are required by statute to be transmitted to Congress.

I was disappointed to see the line in the administration's testimony that they do not stand behind these agreements and hinted towards reopening the painstakingly negotiated products. As we know, we are here today as the result of months of work between FDA and stakeholders to examine the program, figure out what is working and what can work better, and come to an agreement on how the program should be for the next 5 years through a public, drawn-out process.

This process is a long one and the statutory deadline for reauthorization is coming up quickly. Congress has never flirted with neglecting its obligation to reauthorize in a timely and responsible manner. I sincerely hope that this holds true for the sixth reauthorization of PDUFA. Along with the other user fee programs, it must be reauthorized so FDA can do its work and patients maintain access to new therapies without a major disruption in the medical product ecosystem.

PDUFA was first enacted as a way to reduce the time it took FDA to review new drugs and biologics and improve access to medical treatments more quickly. Over the years, the user fees provided under PDUFA have allowed the FDA to hire additional staff and improve the efficiency and predictability of the review process.

Prior to the first PDUFA, the median time for FDA for approval of standard applications was 28 months. Today, the median time for approval for standard applications has been reduced to 12 months, and first-cycle approval rates are at 95 percent. The U.S. remains the gold standard for drug approval and evaluation of safety and efficiency.

The commitment letter for PDUFA VI includes a number of performance goals meant to help the agency with recruiting and retaining the scientific and professional staff needed to keep pace with the science. For the first time, PDUFA VI also includes specified agency hiring goals. This builds on the hiring provisions in the 21st Century Cures that will help the agency to compete with the private sector in terms of competitive salary, and gives the agency the authority to hire scientific and technical staff needed to support medical project review.

There have been some that have criticized FDA for being a barrier to the access to innovative new drugs. This is inaccurate. Contrary to the description by the President and others who want to roll back patient safety measures, the FDA's approval process is not slow and burdensome. Today, more than two-thirds of novel drugs are approved first by the FDA rather than anywhere else in the world.

It is clear that PDUFA has been successful in meeting the goal of improving efficiency of the drug review process at FDA and ensuring patients have access to novel therapies. The policies and goals included in the agreements reflect what these stakeholders value and will help ensure advancements and improvements within the FDA and ultimately health care more broadly.

I want to thank the agency and the stakeholders for their leadership on this agreement that will continue the trajectory of patient-centered innovation at the FDA. 21st Century Cures did a great job to advance such reforms and help get new cures from the lab table to the bedside. I look forward to hearing from the FDA and other witnesses on how this agreement will build on these successes and continue to advance the modern, efficient FDA and a healthy pipeline of medical breakthroughs. And I yield back my time.

Mr. GUTHRIE [presiding]. The gentleman yields back his time.

Mr. GREEN. Do we have any other opening statements? No, OK. Mr. GUTHRIE. We have none on our side. OK, we will turn to the witnesses. We want to thank all of our witnesses for being here today and taking the time to testify before the subcommittee. And each witness will have an opportunity to give an opening statement followed by a round of questions from members.

And we have two panels of witnesses today, and we will begin with our first witness, Dr. Janet Woodcock, Center for Drug Evaluation and Research, Food and Drug Administration. We appreciate you being here. And, Dr. Woodcock, you are now recognized for 5 minutes to give an opening statement.

STATEMENT OF JANET WOODCOCK, M.D., CENTER FOR DRUG EVALUATION AND RESEARCH, FOOD AND DRUG ADMINISTRATION

Dr. Woodcock. Thank you, and thanks to the members of the subcommittee for inviting me to testify at this important hearing. We are talking here about a program that has been going on for 25 years, the prescription drug user fee program. And as result, as we have already heard, over that time U.S. patients have gone from being one of the last in the world to obtain access to new drugs to in most cases being the first patients in the world who can get access to innovative new therapies, all at the same time maintaining the standards that FDA has for safety and effectiveness of these therapies.

At the same time, we have moved from multiple cycle scenario to predominantly first-cycle approval for these drugs, meaning that the industry and FDA have enough communication, the standards are clear enough, they are able to submit a complete application that can be reviewed and approved without further delay. And this is a great time efficiency and resource efficiency for industry for the FDA and for the medical community alike.

Also, this program has allowed us to accommodate the advances in medical science that have occurred recently over the last several decades. Congress and the U.S. investment in NIH and in biomedical research has caused tremendous growth in scientific understanding. Now we are really contemplating, we have approved drugs for example that are antisense oligonucleotides that act directly on people's DNA. We are looking at multiple applications for gene therapies although none have been approved yet. We are looking at multiple cellular therapies that are under development.

And so this promise that you have been hearing about science is really coming about and we have approved cures for various conditions such as hepatitis C, which has long been a scourge of people.

So the next programmatic proposals, the enhancements for the sixth iteration of this, try to build on the accomplishments that we already have. And as has already been said, the first one is really aligned with the Cures legislation that was passed and that is enhancing the ability to capture patient voice in drug development. Not just on benefit-risks, but patients want to tell us what we should study, what matters to them. What do they want ameliorated about their disease? What is most important? How should we study it?

They want to know, they want to tell us how trials should be designed that work for patients. People always wonder why there is so many dropouts in the trials, missing data. Well, because we designed the trials in a way that patients couldn't participate. So the patient voice is critical, and then at the end of the day how much risk are people willing to trade off in uncertainty for the benefits, the potential benefits of any given therapy. And this will require a rigorous process to generate and develop all these data and bring the patients in, in a rigorous way. It is envisioned in Cures and laid out in Cures, and the programmatic enhancements of PDUFA VI would bolster our ability to do that in a timely manner.

Also, there is support for the Breakthrough Therapy Program. Now what I will say about that is that is probably the first program that has really shortened drug development. As we have all said, drug review isn't the problem. It occurs now in a timely manner, predictable manner, based on PDUFA. But drug development is still a very gnarly problem. It takes too long and it costs too much, right, and there are many failures.

Breakthrough has been the first program as actually drug development time has been shortened, and you have heard that before this committee from a number of witnesses, taking several years off of drug development in the overall time it takes to get those drugs. Part of it is the quality of the compounds, the molecules that are developed under and given breakthrough, but also part of it is the support that FDA is willing to give. And so the new program would give additional resources.

There is also, as was envisioned in Cures, support for biomarker qualification also for the better use of surrogate endpoints, an advancement of clinical trial design, something dear to my heart and I would be happy to talk to you about; advances in the use of real world evidence, which is also a Cures theme; better communication with industry to make sure that we are always on the same page and we move things along; and then administrative improvements including oversight of some of the administrative processes, reports, and financial oversight, to make sure the management and planning of the program is as good as it can be.

So I believe this captures in the programmatic proposals many of the modern themes that need to now address improvements in drug development and drug approval, and I would be happy to answer any questions.

[The prepared statement of Dr. Woodcock follows:]

"Examining FDA's Prescription Drug User Fee Program"

Testimony of Janet Woodcock, MD

Director, Center for Drug Evaluation and Research

Before the United States House of Representatives Committee on Energy and Commerce Subcommittee on Health

March 22, 2017

U.S. Department of Health and Human Services

U.S. Food and Drug Administration

www.fda.gov

FDA U.S. FOOD & DRUG ADMINISTRATION

Introduction

Mr. Chairman and Members of the Subcommittee, thank you for the opportunity to testify today on the sixth authorization of the Prescription Drug User Fee Act (PDUFA), also referred to as "PDUFA VI," and the Food and Drug Administration's (FDA or the Agency) efforts to deliver timely access to safe and effective new medications for all Americans.

The PDUFA reauthorization proposal described below was submitted to Congress in December under the previous Administration, and reflects a different approach to the Federal Budget. The Blueprint Budget supports many of the goals of the reauthorization proposal but proposes a different way of financing these goals. The Administration looks forward to working with Congress, with industry input, to develop a reauthorization proposal that speeds the development and approval of vital drugs and biologics that are safe and effective.

PDUFA

The timely review of the safety and effectiveness of new drug applications (NDAs) and biologics license applications (BLAs) is central to FDA's mission to protect and promote the public health – and PDUFA is essential to these efforts.

Before PDUFA's enactment in 1992, Americans' access to innovative, new medicines lagged behind other countries. FDA's premarket review process was understaffed, unpredictable, and slow. The Agency lacked sufficient staff to perform timely reviews or develop procedures and standards to assure a more rigorous, consistent, and predictable process.

To tackle these challenges, Congress passed PDUFA, which authorized FDA to collect industry user fees to hire additional staff and upgrade its information technology systems. In return, it committed the Agency to speed the application review process for new drugs without compromising its high standards for new drug safety, efficacy, and quality.

Speeding Americans' Access to Safe and Effective New Therapies

PDUFA has revolutionized the United States' drug approval process. It reversed the lag in drug approvals that prompted its creation, providing Americans with more rapid access to safe and effective new drugs and biologics.

As shown in Figure 1, today, almost two-thirds of new active substances approved in the world market are launched first in the United States. To put this figure in perspective, that is more than triple the rate approved first in the United States in the first year of PDUFA.

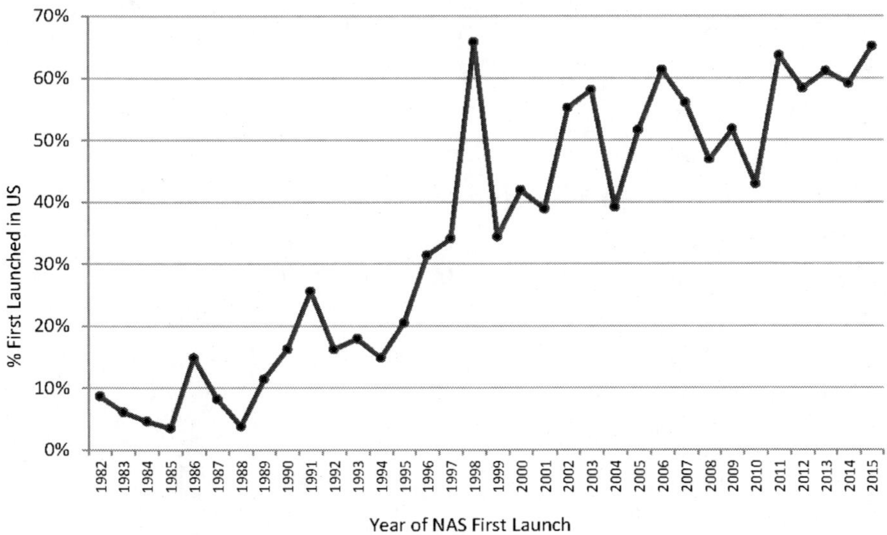

Source: *Scrip Magazine* (1982 - 2006), *Pharmaprojects/Citeline* Pharma R&D Annual Review (2007 - 2016)

Figure 1. US Share of New Active Substances (NAS) Launched on the World Market.

The five-year reauthorization cycles for PDUFA have supported continuous program innovation, evaluation, and improvement. The enhancements to the process of human drug review originally focused on the FDA pre-market review of NDAs and BLAs. Through successive PDUFA reauthorizations, program enhancements have evolved and expanded to include extensive communication and consultation between drug sponsors and FDA throughout drug development. This has enabled better incorporation of advances in regulatory science applied to drug development and regulatory oversight. The continued modernization of drug review under PDUFA has also strengthened and enabled innovation in approaches to post-market safety. Most recently, the program has been enhanced by increasing patient focus and modernizing supporting informatics.

These enhancements have contributed to the United States becoming a global leader in drug innovation and Americans are typically the first to benefit from safe and effective new medicines. PDUFA, with its reauthorization cycles, has resulted in a scientifically and financially strong program with transparent stakeholder engagement as a routine way of doing business.

Throughout this program evolution, FDA has continued to review large volumes of sponsor submissions and deliver predictably high levels of performance against PDUFA goal commitments for timely regulatory review and development phase consultation, as shown in Figure 2, below.

Increasing the Timeliness and Efficiency of Premarket Review

A key element of the success of the PDUFA program is ongoing development-phase consultation provided to drug sponsors by FDA, helping to minimize unnecessary or suboptimal development steps, and getting important new drugs to patients more rapidly and efficiently. FDA's capacity to provide sponsors, including small first-time innovators, with timely advice enabled by PDUFA funding, has contributed to the strong drug development pipeline in the United States today. This is reflected in the increased numbers of drug development programs underway in companies, and the corresponding growth in company requests for development phase meetings with FDA, as shown in Figure 3.

The volume of formal meetings requested by drug sponsors has steadily grown over the course of PDUFA. Early and frequent communication between sponsors and FDA serves to improve the efficiency of drug development. Indeed, it is one of the cornerstones of the Breakthrough Therapy program. FDA-sponsor meetings help sponsors navigate key milestones during drug development, support the assembly and submission of sponsors' marketing applications, and enable sponsors to clarify requirements for complete application submissions and potentially avoid the need for an additional review cycle.

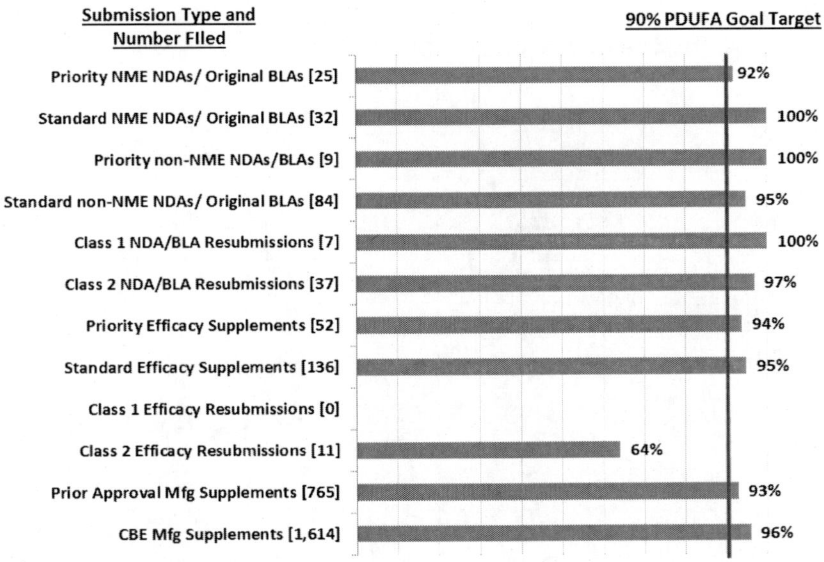

Data as of 9/30/2016

Figure 2. FDA Review Performance - FY 2015: Percent of Submissions Acted on by Goal Date[1].

The improvement in the quality of drug development programs and the submitted applications, supported by these PDUFA-enabled consultations

[1] NME = New Molecular Entity; NDA = New Drug Application; BLA = Biologic Licensing Application; CBE = Changes-Being-Effected

between FDA and drug sponsors, is but one explanation for the observed trend toward higher first cycle approvals of applications for novel drugs (referred to as new molecular entity (NME) NDAs and BLAs), as shown in Figure 4.

Development-phase consultations can be particularly helpful in support of the most innovative drug programs. Of the NME NDAs and BLAs that FDA approved in calendar year 2016, over one-third were indicated for rare diseases. In addition, over one-third (36 percent) of the drugs approved by the Center for Drug Evaluation and Research were first in their drug class and over eighty percent (86 percent) were approved first in the United States.

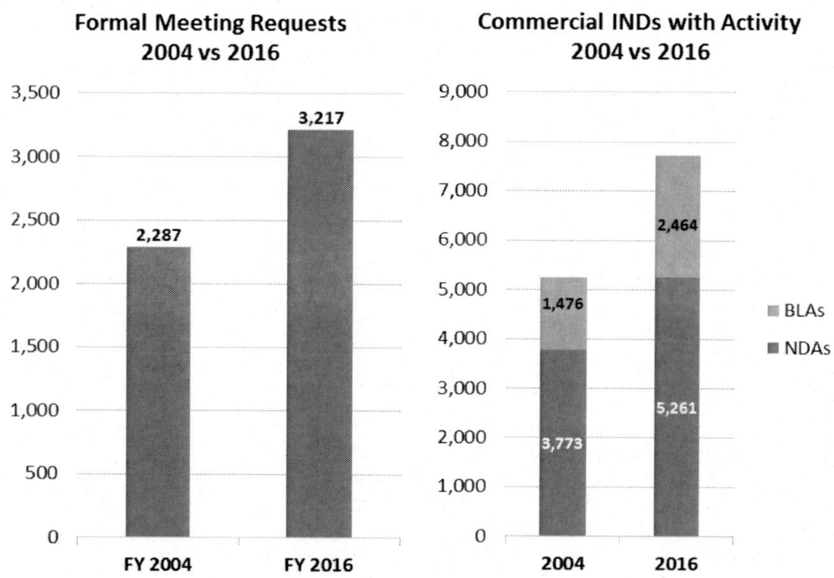

- IND Data represents a 12 month Academic period of July 1st-June 30th
- Activity is defined as any incoming submissions received within the reporting period on/after the date of the new IND application.
- Meeting Data as of 9/30/2016.
- Data includes activity for both FDA's Center for Drug Evaluation and Research and Center for Biologics Evaluation and Research.

Figure 3. FDA Commercial Investigational New Drug (INDs) with Activity and Formal Meeting Requests 2004 vs. 2016.

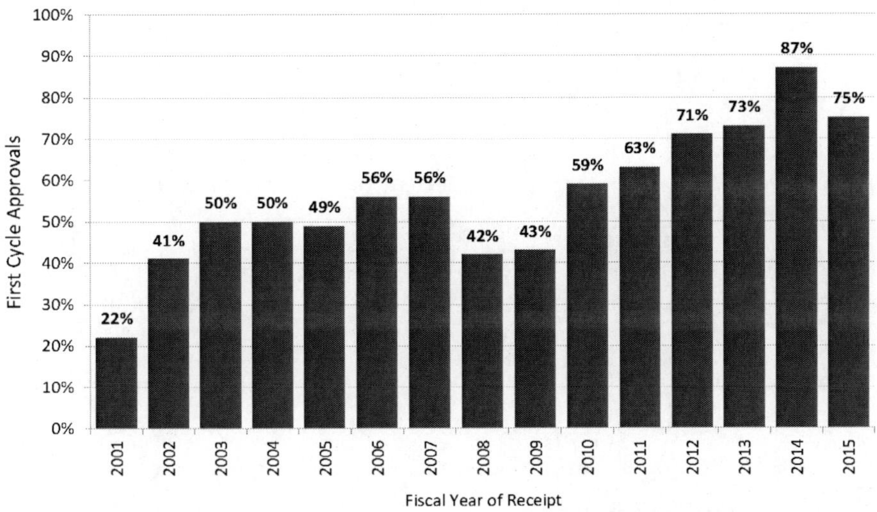

- Multiple applications pertaining to single new molecular/biologic entity (e.g., single ingredient and combinations) are only counted once. Therefore, the numbers represented here for filings are not indicate of workload in the PDUFA V Program.
- Original BLAs that do not contain a new active ingredient are excluded. Percentages exclude pending applications from the denominator.
- Data includes activity for both FDA's Center for Drug Evaluation and Research and Center for Biologics Evaluation and Research.

Figure 4. FDA NME NDA/BLA First Action Approval Rate.

While a standard review is typically completed in ten months, FDA expedites review for priority drugs to be completed within six months. Priority drugs are generally targeted at severe illnesses with few or no available therapeutic options. They typically receive greater assistance from FDA reviewers throughout the development process, including providing advice in the design and implementation of the clinical trials necessary to demonstrate product safety and effectiveness.

In 2016, over 60 percent of NME NDAs and new BLAs approved by FDA benefited from one or more of FDA's expedited programs.

Expanded Access to Investigational Products

While the best means of providing access to useful medical treatments for all Americans is to approve drugs demonstrated to be safe and effective as quickly as possible, FDA also recognizes circumstances in which there may be value to patients and physicians in having access to products prior to marketing approval. In some cases where an individual has a serious or life- threatening disease and lacks a satisfactory therapy, that individual may believe that a promising but not yet fully evaluated treatment is his or her best choice.

FDA allows for access to investigational products through clinical trials and the Agency's Expanded Access program. Clinical trials collect the necessary clinical information needed for FDA review and, if appropriate, approval, of investigational drugs, thereby making the drug widely available to patients. However, there are times when an individual cannot enroll in a clinical trial. In these cases, the patient may be able to gain access to an investigational therapy through the Expanded Access program.

In order for an individual patient to qualify for the Expanded Access program, several criteria must be met, including that the patient must have a serious or life-threatening disease or condition and no comparable or satisfactory alternative therapy. The patient's physician then approaches the pharmaceutical company to ask for its agreement that it will provide the drug being sought. The company has the right to approve or disapprove the physician's request. If the company agrees to the physician's request, the physician can then apply to FDA for authorization to proceed. Should they do so, they are highly likely to be allowed to proceed with the expanded access use. FDA has authorized more than 99 percent of the requests received in Fiscal Years 2010-2015. Emergency requests are usually granted immediately over the phone and non-emergencies are processed in a median of four days.

Access to investigational products requires the active cooperation of the treating physician, industry and FDA in order to be successful. In particular, the company developing the investigational product must be willing to provide it – FDA cannot force a company to manufacture a product or to make a product available. Companies might have their own reasons to turn down requests for their investigational products, including their desire to maintain their clinical development program or simply because they have not produced enough of the product.

For over 20 years, FDA has been committed to ensuring that this program works well for patients and has recently made significant improvements to its functioning and efficiency.

Breakthrough Therapy Designation

The Breakthrough Therapy (BT) program, authorized by the FDA Safety and Innovation Act (FDASIA), has further enhanced the engagement of FDA and sponsors during drug development. This program, which is for new drugs to treat serious and life-threatening diseases with unmet medical need, calls for intensive FDA-sponsor consultation during development, when preliminary clinical evidence indicates that the drug may demonstrate substantial improvement over available therapies on one or more clinically significant endpoints.

Given the known benefits of development-phase consultation with FDA, the BT designation has been much sought after by sponsors. As of November 30, 2016, FDA had received 492 requests for BT designation and had granted 165 requests. Figure 5 shows the trend of increasing numbers of development programs.

Although oncology, hematology and antiviral products account for the largest share of BT designation requests in CDER, it should be noted that BT requests and the granted designations and ongoing programs span the entire spectrum of disease areas as shown in Figure 6a, reflecting granted designations as of November 30, 2016. In CBER, most of the BT designation requests and granted designations are for gene therapies, vaccines and immunotherapies as shown in Figure 6b.

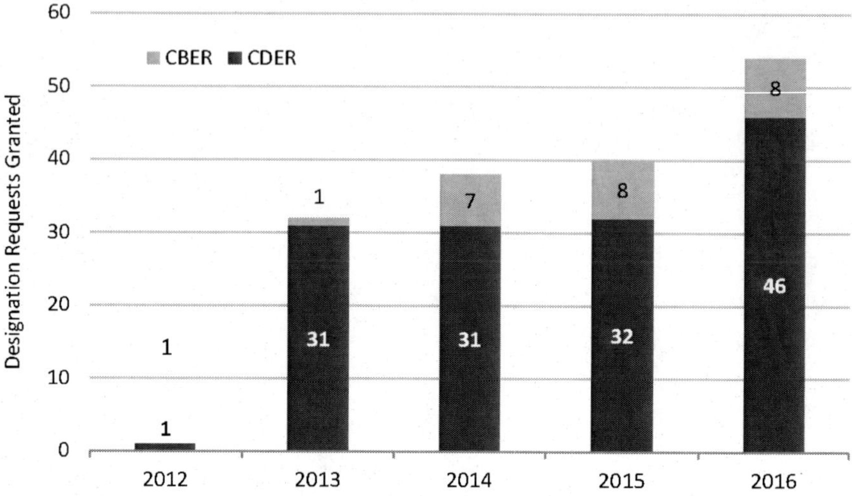

Figure 5. Number of FDA Breakthrough Designated Development Programs by Fiscal Year of Designation.

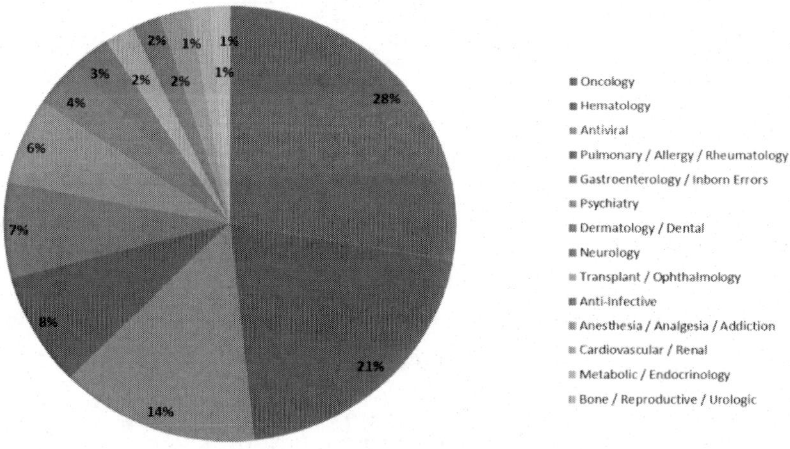

Figure 6a. CDER Breakthrough Therapy Requests Granted by Product Type.

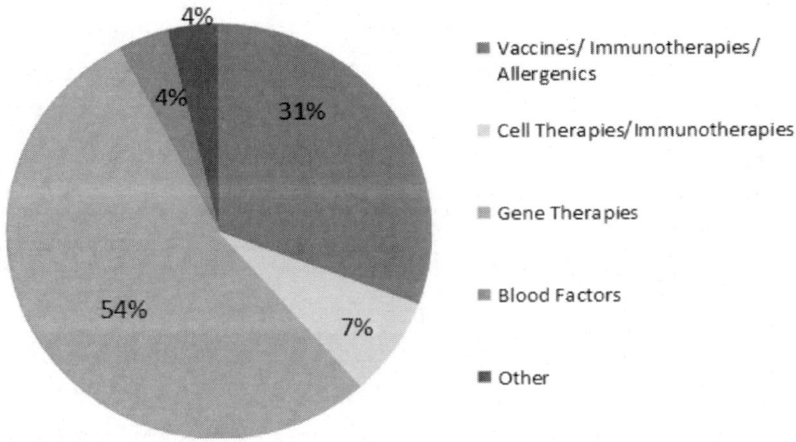

Data as of 12/1/16. Figures include total # of granted breakthrough designations for drug/indications under active IND development but have not yet received marketing approval or rescission decision.

Figure 6b. CBER Breakthrough Therapy Requests Granted by Product Type.

PDUFA V

We are currently in the final year of the PDUFA V program. Over the years since the start of PDUFA I in 1992, the complexity of scientific and clinical issues in the study of new drugs has grown, including use of genetic targeting, biomarkers, novel trial designs, plans and programs to ensure effective post-market risk management. These approaches and issues were less common or nonexistent at the start of PDUFA. In addition, predictability and increased communication with FDA during drug development and application review emerged as a top priority for drug sponsors.

PDUFA V sought to achieve a better balance between the desire for increased communication with sponsors and the need to ensure adequate review time for the most complex and innovative products reviewed by FDA. This resulted in a cornerstone of the PDUFA V agreement, a new program for NME NDAs and BLA reviews that is designed to promote greater transparency and improve communication between the FDA review team and the applicant. We anticipated that the increased communications before application submissions and at key points within the first review cycle would ensure that FDA had access to all of the information that might inform and enable a first-cycle approval for those applications that could be approved, avoiding unnecessary additional cycles of review. This would enable faster access to new drugs for the patients who need them and would help reduce avoidable costs for drug sponsors.

A key measure of program success is the percentage of applications approved in a single, first review cycle. Figure 7 illustrates the success of the PDUFA V NME Program in achieving its first cycle review goals for both standard and priority reviews. The figure presents the share of first-cycle approvals for priority and standard NDAs and BLAs filed. First cycle approvals for NME NDAs and new BLAs have been significantly higher under the new PDUFA V review program.

Other PDUFA V enhancements include improved communications during drug development, strengthening the rare disease program, exploring new methods for regulatory science, and implementation of structured benefit-risk assessment. PDUFA V also provided for additional drug safety enhancements focused on standardizing the design of Risk Evaluation and Management Systems (REMS) and using the Sentinel Initiative, FDA's active surveillance systems for post-market safety (see PDUFA IV), to evaluate drug safety issues. This has prepared the way for expanded reliance on the data from Sentinel.

Patient-Focused Drug Development

As part of the PDUFA V benefit-risk assessment initiative, FDA and industry recognized that patients are uniquely positioned to inform aspects of FDA's benefit-risk assessment, particularly the understanding of the disease and its severity and the adequacy of existing treatment options. Therefore, FDA committed to hold at least 20 public meetings over the five year period, with each meeting focused on obtaining direct patient input in a specific disease area. This initiative, referred to as "patient-focused drug development," has since been described as potentially transformational in advancing the role of the patient in drug development and decision-making. Although initially committing to conduct 20 meetings, FDA is on track to conduct 24 meetings each in different disease areas. The goal of the meeting is to hear from patients and their caregivers about the impact of their disease on their lives, and for FDA to hear more about what treatment benefits would be most meaningful to patients, and what treatment burdens are most important to consider. Following each meeting FDA develops a *Voice of the Patient* report to capture what was heard in the meetings (and comments from patients received in the docket); these documents serve as a valuable reference for FDA reviewers in subsequent drug reviews and related decision making.

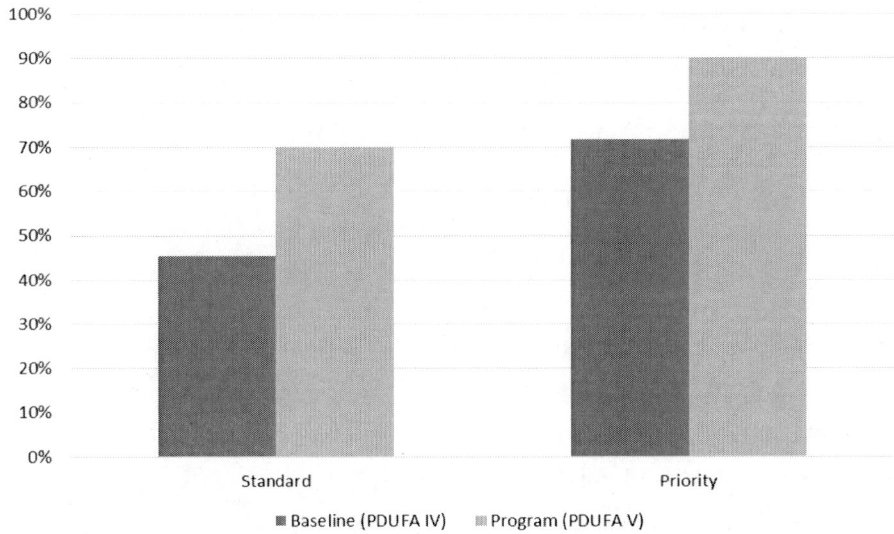

Data includes activity for both FDA's Center for Drug Evaluation and Research and Center for Biologics Evaluation and Research.

Figure 7. Findings of the Final Assessment of the PDUFA V NME Review Program

Patient-focused drug development has provided key learnings for FDA that are being carried forward and integrated into our methods and approaches to development and decision making. We recognize that patients with chronic serious disease are experts on what it is like to live with their condition, and we have learned that they want to be as active as possible in the work to develop and evaluate new treatments. In the past, patients' "chief complaints" were often not factored explicitly into drug development plans (as endpoints and measures of drug benefit planned in trials), and this is an area of needed attention going forward. Although the PDUFA V patient-focused drug development initiative was intended as a pilot to elicit broader patient input, a key question for the agency was how to best build upon this pilot to advance the science and processes for effective incorporation of the patient's voice in drug development and decision making.

In preparing for PDUFA VI reauthorization discussions, FDA has worked to build on the successes and learnings of PDUFA V and pursue new areas of opportunity for innovation in the enhancement of regulatory decision tools and new potential sources of evidence to inform drug development and review.

PDUFA VI Reauthorization Process

Congress directed the Agency to reach out to all stakeholders to solicit thoughts and insights on PDUFA reauthorization and changes to PDUFA performance goals. FDA held an initial public meeting on July 15, 2015, which included presentations by FDA and representatives of different stakeholder groups, including patient advocates, consumer groups, regulated industry, health professionals, and academic researchers. A transcript and Webcast recording are available on FDA's website at https://www.fda.gov/ForIndustry/UserFees/PrescriptionDrugUserFee/ucm446608.htm.

Based on comments to a public docket, and the Agency's own internal analyses of program challenge areas, FDA developed a set of potential proposed enhancements for PDUFA VI and began negotiations with industry. Parallel discussions with public stakeholders were held monthly from September 2015—February 2016 to update participants on ongoing negotiations and solicit thoughts. Meeting minutes were posted on FDA's website and are available at https://www.fda.gov/ForIndustry/UserFees/PrescriptionDrugUserFee/ucm446608.htm.

A final public meeting was held on August 15, 2016, to discuss the PDUFA VI agreement and engage with interested parties on proposed recommendations. A summary of the agreement and a draft of the Commitment Letter were provided a month in advance of this discussion.

Final PDUFA VI recommendations were transmitted to Congress in December 2016.

PDUFA VI Overview

Building on the success of previous agreements, PDUFA VI continues to support early and meaningful communication between FDA and drug sponsors to deliver safe and effective medications to Americans more quickly, and, expands on such communications by providing resources for the popular, highly successful, and resource-intensive Breakthrough Therapy program and streamlining review of products combining a drug or biologic with a device. It enhances drug development tools including biomarker qualification and provides resources to increase our understanding of how "real-world evidence" can be generated and used appropriately in regulatory decision making. The agreement also enables us to leverage the use of real-world health data by enhancing the capabilities of FDA's Sentinel System.

Many of these core provisions are explained in greater detail below.

Capturing the Patient Voice in Drug Development

Central to PDUFA VI, and its largest single investment component, are plans to elevate patient voices in developing new drugs to treat their diseases. The agreement shares the Committee's goals reflected in the 21st Century Cures Act ("Cures") – and the highest priority of our stakeholders – to leverage essential patient input and insights to fight disease.

We are building on the success of PDUFA V which established the Patient-Focused Drug Development (PFDD) program to obtain valuable patient perspectives. Areas of focus were carefully chosen based on a public process soliciting patient and stakeholder input. Under PDUFA VI, we look forward to engaging in a transparent, multi-stakeholder approach that will lead to development of the methods and approaches to ensure patients not only become active participants but informants to industry drug development and agency review. The performance commitments and matching resources to sufficiently staff this critical new work are intended to bridge from patient-focused drug development meetings to fit-for-purpose tools to collect meaningful patient input, including capturing information on the natural progression of disease.

To help identify sound and rigorous methods to capture science-based, disease-specific patient input, FDA has committed to enhance its staff capacity, hold a series of four public workshops, and develop four key guidance documents on needed methods and approaches. The Agency will also publish on its website a repository of publicly available tools as a resource for stakeholders and ongoing efforts.

We are gratified by the enthusiastic response within the patient community to PFDD, and look forward to working with the broader community to advance the science of patient input – and deliver new and better treatment options.

Building a Solid Foundation for Breakthrough Therapies

The Breakthrough Therapy program, authorized by FDASIA, has become one of the most popular components of the human drug review program with requests and designations far exceeding expectations.

The increase in promising new drugs to treat serious and life-threatening diseases with unmet medical need is, of course, a very good thing for both patients and public health. But the growth of the BT program has strained limited available review staff resources. A hallmark of the BT program is intensive Agency interaction with sponsors during the development process on complex products with transformative potential. This "all hands on deck" approach provides a sponsor of a designated breakthrough product with guidance from the Agency on efficient drug development beginning as early as the Phase I period, an organizational commitment to involve senior managers, and eligibility for rolling review. Many of the BT designations granted so far have been for rare disease indications.

The PDUFA VI agreement provides dedicated funding to ensure the sustained success of the BT program. Additional resources will enable FDA to increase review staff and to supplement resources for clinical pharmacology, statistics, and product quality. This renewed commitment will enable the Agency to continue to work closely with sponsors to ensure expedited development and review of breakthrough therapies for serious or life-threatening diseases.

Advancing Biomarker Development

FDA and industry share the goals of Cures to accelerate development of reliable biomarkers to advance important new therapies. Biomarkers are currently used throughout the drug development process, including as surrogate endpoints to support earlier evidence for regulatory decision-making when evidence from a clinical endpoint could take much longer or require many more patients to be studied.

FDA commonly uses surrogate endpoints in accelerated approvals where confirmatory evidence is required to verify the expected clinical benefit after marketing begins. Surrogate endpoints have been the basis for 60 percent of rare-disease approvals. Once a surrogate endpoint is well established to predict clinical benefit, surrogate endpoints can be used to support traditional approvals as well. For example, FDA regularly relies on a surrogate endpoint for approval of new therapies for diabetes (the HbA1C test, a measurement of hemoglobin with attached sugar in the blood that reflects the extent and persistence of elevated blood sugar) greatly expanding patient treatment options.

The PDUFA VI proposed enhancements include some of the same activities specified in Cures. PDUFA VI addressed the opportunity for application of biomarkers in two different areas, one involving proprietary use of a biomarker as a surrogate endpoint in a specific drug development program, and the other involving the more public process of biomarker qualification as a drug development tool.

FDA recognizes that early consultation can be important to an efficient development program when a sponsor intends to use a biomarker as a new surrogate endpoint that has never been used as the primary basis for product approval in the proposed context of use. The PDUFA VI commitments therefore provide for early consultation with the sponsor to enable the FDA review team to consult with senior management to evaluate the sponsor's proposal before providing advice to the sponsor on a critical aspect of their development program. This will enable FDA to discuss the feasibility of the surrogate as a primary endpoint, any knowledge gaps, and how these gaps should be addressed before the surrogate endpoint could be used as the primary basis for approval.

PDUFA VI also provides enhancements for the more public drug development tool qualification pathway for biomarkers. The biomarker qualification program was established to support FDA's work with external partners to develop biomarkers that aid in the drug development process. To facilitate the enhancement of the drug development tools qualification pathway for biomarkers in PDUFA VI, FDA proposes to convene a public meeting to discuss taxonomy and a framework with standards for biomarkers used in drug development, to develop guidance on biomarker taxonomy, contexts of uses, and general evidentiary standards for biomarker qualification, and to maintain a public website to communicate a list of biomarker qualification submissions in the qualification process.

Meaningful progress in developing additional biomarkers for public qualification requires collaboration among a wide range of stakeholders. FDA will continue to work with the National Institutes of Health, the Biomarkers Consortium, the Critical Path Institute and others to advance biomarker development.

Streamlining Combination Product Review

More streamlined oversight of combination products is another FDA and industry priority reflected in PDUFA VI. Under the proposed enhancements FDA will pursue improvements in inter-center and intra-center combination product review coordination and transparency for PDUFA products that are combination products regulated by CDER and CBER (PDUFA combination products). FDA proposes to enhance staff capacity and capability across the relevant medical product centers and the Office of Combination Products to more efficiently, effectively, and consistently review combination products. FDA also proposes to streamline the process for combination product review and to improve the Agency's ability to track combination product review workload, including a third party assessment of current practices for combination drug product review.

Our goal, consistent with Cures, is to enhance the overall efficiency, consistency, and predictability of combination product review without imposing new administrative burdens.

Under PDUFA VI enhancements FDA will also establish new performance goals and submission procedures for the review of human factors protocols for PDUFA combination products. These goals will be to provide the sponsor with written comments on these protocols within 60 days of receipt. The goals to provide written comments within 60 days will begin at the 50 percent level in FY 2019, and increase to 90 percent by FY 2021.

Advancing the Use of Complex Innovative Trial Designs and Model Informed Drug Development

FDA routinely works closely with industry to facilitate innovative approaches to drug development that maintain our high standards for drug safety and efficacy. PDUFA VI promises to encourage future efforts by advancing Model-Informed Drug Development (MIDD) and the use of complex innovative and adaptive clinical trial designs.

The development and application of exposure-based, biological, and statistical models derived from preclinical and clinical data sources can be used to inform regulatory decision making, for example, in determining patient selection in clinical trials, individualized dosing for specific populations, or the need for post-marketing studies. To facilitate the development and application of these approaches during PDUFA VI, FDA proposes to convene a series of workshops to identify best practices for MIDD, to conduct a pilot program, to develop guidance on MIDD, and to update policies and procedures, as appropriate, to incorporate guidelines for the evaluation of MIDD approaches.

To facilitate the advancement and use of complex adaptive, Bayesian, and other novel clinical trial designs during PDUFA VI, FDA proposes to convene a public workshop on complex innovative trial designs, publish guidance on complex innovative trial designs, to conduct a pilot program, and to update policies and procedures as appropriate to incorporate guidelines on evaluating complex innovative trial designs.

Utilizing Real-World Observational Data

It has been said that medical care and biomedical research are in the midst of a data revolution, and networked systems, electronic health records, electronic insurance claims databases, social media, patient registries, and other new sources may comprise an immense new set of sources for data about health and healthcare. In addition, these "real-world" sources can provide data about patients in the setting of their environments—whether at home or at work—and in the social context of their lives. There is little doubt that the new sources of data now becoming increasingly available to researchers, clinicians, and patients hold enormous potential for improving the quality, safety, and efficiency of medical care. More work is needed to understand both the promise and pitfalls of far-reaching technological changes, including the multiple dimensions of quality and fitness for purpose for appropriate use of such data in regulatory decision making.

FDA recognizes the potential value of utilizing "real-world" evidence in evaluating not only the safety of medications but also their effectiveness. To better understand how real-world evidence can be generated and used appropriately in product evaluation, FDA proposes to conduct one or more public workshops, as well as other appropriate activities (e.g., pilot studies or methodology development projects). Considering the available input, FDA will then publish draft guidance on how real-world evidence can contribute to the assessment of safety and effectiveness in regulatory submissions.

Under PDUFA VI, FDA also proposes to pursue a more well-established use of real-world evidence to support post market drug safety surveillance utilizing Sentinel. FDA's Sentinel Initiative is a long-term program designed to build and implement a national electronic system for monitoring the safety of FDA-approved medical products. FDA recently transitioned from the Mini-Sentinel pilot to the Sentinel System, but full utilization of the Sentinel System remains a work in progress. Continued development and integration of the Sentinel System is needed to realize the system's full value to the postmarketing safety review process.

To help realize the full value of the Sentinel System during PDUFA VI, FDA proposes to continue to expand the systems' data sources and core capabilities, to systematically integrate Sentinel into postmarketing review activities, to enhance communication practices with sponsors and the public regarding general methodologies for Sentinel queries, and to conduct an analysis of the impact of Sentinel expansion and integration for regulatory purposes.

Hiring and Retaining Highly Qualified Experts

To speed and improve development of safe and effective new therapies for patients requires that FDA hire and retain sufficient numbers and types of technical and scientific experts to efficiently conduct reviews of human drug applications. In order to strengthen this core function during PDUFA VI, FDA proposes to commit to completing implementation of: a modernized position management system, corporate recruiting practices, augmenting capacity with contractor support, a dedicated scientific recruiting function, metric goals for human drug review staff hiring, and a comprehensive independent assessment of hiring and retention system performance. We want to thank you again for providing vital new hiring authority in Cures. Cures will greatly improve FDA's ability to hire and retain scientific experts in more complex and specialized areas and meet our growing responsibilities.

The hiring commitments proposed in PDUFA VI will complement Cures by supplementing the expertise and resources the Agency needs to perform its vital prescription drug mission.

Enhancing Management of User Fee Resources

FDA is committed to enhancing management of PDUFA resources and ensuring PDUFA user fee resources are administered, allocated, and reported in an efficient and transparent manner. In PDUFA VI, the Agency proposes to establish a resource capacity planning function to improve its ability to analyze current resource needs and project future resource needs, modernize its time reporting approach, conduct an evaluation of PDUFA program resource management, and publish a five-year PDUFA financial plan with annual updates.

In addition, under PDUFA VI, FDA proposes to enhance the program fee structure and related mechanisms, to achieve increased predictability, stability, and efficiency. The current overall PDUFA fee structure and the fee setting process were established in 1992. Both FDA and industry recognize that updating some elements of the fee structure and the fee setting process will enhance administrative efficiency and the predictability and stability of fee amounts and revenues and improve FDA's ability to engage in long-term financial planning. FDA proposes to shift a greater proportion of the target revenue allocation to more predictable fee-paying types (20 percent to applications; 80 percent to Program fees), and make other modifications to improve efficiency and stability including discontinuation of the establishment and supplement fees, modifying the annual fee billing date to minimize the need for multiple billing cycles, and other technical changes.

Conclusion

PDUFA has revolutionized the drug review process in the United States, allowing FDA to speed the application review process without compromising the Agency's high standards. User fees offer a strong example of what can be achieved when FDA, industry, and other stakeholders work together towards the same goal. User fees provide a critical way to ensure that FDA has the resources needed to conduct reviews in a timely fashion. While we have made demonstrable progress in partnering to bring drug and biologics to market in as timely a manner as possible, we know that more work remains to be done to further enhance and optimize our processes. The reauthorization of PDUFA will allow FDA to build upon the program's demonstrated success, and in so doing, further benefit patients and affirm our nation's standing as a global leader in biomedical innovation.

Mr. Guthrie. Thank you. I want to thank you for your testimony. We will now move to the first Q&A portion of the hearing, and I will begin the questioning and recognize myself for 5 minutes.

So Dr. Woodcock, as part of 21st Century Cures, this committee included provisions that set up FDA Intercenter Institutes of Excellence in major disease areas to improve coordination across the agency. FDA has since established the Oncology Center of Excellence. Can you provide us with an update on how things are going so far and if there is anything we can do to help ensure smooth and timely implementation?

Dr. WOODCOCK. Yes. The Oncology Center of Excellence is considered a joint venture by the three medical products centers, Center for Biologics, Center for Devices and Radiological Health, and Center for Drugs. And so we put this together jointly, it resides up in the office right above us. Dr. Richard Pazdur is the director of that office.

And the procedures that we are running, they will review the clinical oncology, the medical oncology portion of any product that comes in with a medical oncology indication to any of the three centers. So they will do the medical part of that review, and Rick will direct it, but it will include oncologists from Drugs and Biologics as appropriate to that particular cancer area.

So we have worked out the procedures and so forth and we expect those applications then will go before the Oncologic Drugs Advisory Committee and be heard. And then the Center, whichever Center has the product, will complete the rest of the product review which is about the quality of the product and the control of that quality, and then we will actually approve the application using the clinical recommendations from the Oncology Center of Excellence.

And the Center also will be the outfacing, outward facing group that will interact with the medical oncology and patient community.

Mr. Guthrie. OK, thank you. I want to yield time to my good friend from Virginia, Mr. Griffith.

Mr. Griffith. Thank you very much. I appreciate that. Dr. Woodcock, prior to the FDA's encouraging the development of abuse deterrent opioids, manufacturers should be incorporating these technologies into their products and testing whether they deter various routes of potential abuse, intranasal, intravenous, et cetera. If they do, manufacturers need to be able to include this data in their product labeling and communicate this useful information to healthcare providers.

I understand a recent exclusivity determination by FDA calls into question whether multiple manufacturers in the same product class could make such claims even if their data justifies it and even if they are using different technologies. Is that accurate?

Dr. Woodcock. It is likely accurate. I think like many of the laws governing exclusivity that Congress passed long ago, they certainly didn't foresee some of the situations. And we struggle all the time with trying to figure out how to apply exclusivity fairly and justly to everyone and yet not disadvantage public health goals that we may have.

Mr. Griffith. And so you would agree it probably would discourage a manufacturer if they can't go forward and discuss that; a company or a manufacturer might not invest as much if they think that somebody has beaten them to the punch by a few months. And so what you are recommending, if I understood your previous answer is, is that we probably should take a look at it and change the law?

Dr. Woodcock. Well, I can't go that far because of course that is your purview.

Mr. Griffith. Yes, ma'am. Thank you.

Dr. Woodcock. But I do believe that times have changed.

Mr. Griffith. Yes, ma'am. I appreciate that. Speaking of product manufacturers being able to share useful scientific data and information about their products with doctors, I understand that some previous leaders at the Department of Health and Human Services would not allow FDA to work with Congress to clarify in a responsible and constitutionally sound manner how manufacturers can communicate truthful and non-misleading off-label information.

Now as you and I were just discussing, I prefer that Congress work with you all to make the rules as opposed to leaving it to the courts to decipher. Will you commit to working with us to set up some clear rules of the road so folks know what they can communicate and what they can't?

Dr. Woodcock. Certainly. We will work with the administration, through the administration with you on this issue.

Mr. Griffith. All right, I appreciate that very much.

With that Mr. Chairman, I appreciate the time and I yield back.

Mr. Guthrie. I yield back my time and I recognize Mr. Green for 5 minutes to ask questions.

Mr. Green. Thank you, Mr. Chairman. And thank you, Dr. Woodcock, again for being here this morning. As I mentioned in my opening statement, I was disappointed to see the line in the administration's testimony that they do not stand behind these agreements and hinted toward a reopening of painstakingly negotiated products. Can you explain to the committee what would happen should Congress fail to reauthorize PDUFA and the other user fees before the statutory deadline in September?

Dr. Woodcock. If there is not a reauthorization, we must initiate our reduction in force process where we would prepare to let go of for the Center for Drugs is maybe 70 percent of the staff working on the process of review in new human drugs. And we do have carryover balance within the user fee agreements that we are supposed to hold some money back. In case the program terminates we can, over several months, have an orderly process to let go of the staff. And that we would have to start thinking about that in July because there are complicated personnel rules that have to do with who has to be notified first and so forth.

Mr. Green. OK, thank you. There seems to be a misunderstanding about the drug development process. We hear often that new therapies take about 10 years to develop and some seem to think that means the application languishes at the agency for a decade. In fact, the FDA review is the final step in the development process and more efficient than ever.

Can you explain to this committee how PDUFA VI builds on the past successes of the program and helps the agency work with stakeholders to not be a bottleneck but a strong partner in getting these new treatments to patients in need?

Dr. Woodcock. Certainly. Obviously we have prioritization programs for breakthrough drugs and for priority drugs where they are reviewed in shorter times. We have gotten some reviews out in 3 months, and a drug approved and on the market after the application is submitted where it is a breakthrough.

So, but that doesn't mean that the development time is short. The development time still is quite long and the failure rate of drugs in development is still very high. Perhaps in some areas nine out of ten drugs that get into human testing fail during human testing at huge cost. So a lot of the efforts we are working on, I believe patient focused drug development, the innovative clinical trials, the surrogate endpoints, and biomarkers, all of which are encompassed in the proposed programmatic changes, will help with this drug development phase and making it as short as possible.

As I said, the Breakthrough Therapy Program has actually worked and some of those development programs in the clinic have only been a couple years, so the time to patients has been shortened dramatically.

Mr. Green. Can you explain to this committee how PDUFA VI builds on the successes of the program in the past and helps the agency work with stakeholders to not be a bottleneck but a strong partner in getting new treatments to the patients in need? Or that is my question. OK, let me get to the next one.

Many provisions of the user fee agreements resemble ideas we advanced in Cures, things like biomarker qualification programs, incorporation of the patient perspective in decision making, and the advancement of innovative clinical trials are goals we have shared. I am concerned about the impact that the administration's proposed hiring freeze would have on FDA, and could it be made hard to advance these shared goals?

User fees under PDUFA also assist the FDA in hiring and retaining staff necessary to support the activities associated with review of drug applications. The commitment letter for PDUFA VI includes a number of performance goals meant to help the agency with recruiting and retaining the scientific professional staff needed to keep pace with science. In fact, for the first time, PDUFA VI also includes specific agency hiring goals. This builds off the hiring provisions in the 21st Century Cures.

Can you discuss further how the PDUFA VI will help the FDA to hire and train the scientific technical workforce needed to fulfill the goals agreed to in the commitment letter?

Dr. Woodcock. Well, for really the first time, this programmatic proposal in PDUFA VI really focuses on some of the administrative processes and tries to set in place some oversight over hiring and so forth, and some new scientific recruitment staff and so forth that would enable us to hire scientists. As I said, the science has really come along, and so we are talking about really high-tech kind of treatments in humans, such as gene therapy in humans and so forth, and we need the scientific staff that are qualified to evaluate those and make sure they are safe as well as that they work.

Mr. Green. Well, my time is almost up. And I know our goal is to make sure you have the resources to do it quicker and not lay in another level of bureaucracy to make it even longer. Thank you, Mr. Chairman.

Mr. Guthrie. Thank you. The gentleman yields back. Mr. Upton is recognized for 5 minutes.

Mr. Upton. Well, thank you, Dr. Woodcock. It is great to see you again, and I know all of us on both sides of the aisle here really appreciated your work and your input from the very beginning on getting 21st Century Cures ultimately to the President. And we knew that by expediting the approval of drugs and devices we were going to need require you all at the FDA to help us and to help chart that course for us and provide the right resources so that you would be able to do your job.

And obviously PDUFA VI is very important, very important. And alarming of course to us, a good message to us is if we don't get it done by summer or show that we have made progress by July and August, certainly by September, that you would actually have to RIF 70 percent of the staff, is quite alarming and ought to serve as turning up the burner for us to get our job done, as we have in the past in a very strong bipartisan way, ultimately getting this bill to the President.

A question for you, Diana DeGette and I sent a letter a couple weeks ago to OMB asking about the federal hiring freeze that the President announced as it relates to the implementation of 21st Century Cures. And of course as you know we came up with offsets, dollar for dollar matching to help with the half billion dollar increase that we gave for the FDA.

Yesterday, it is my understanding that you told the Senate Health Committee—and I have to again compliment Lamar Alexander and the great work that they did over there. But yesterday you told the Health Committee that the White House did give the FDA permission to move forward with hiring on the select user fee positions needed to implement Cures. I don't know if that is a quote or not, but that is my understanding.

Can you provide some more detail? We have not heard back. It is my understanding we have not heard back from our letter that we sent to the White House, but can you tell us more details about the type of hiring that is going to be needed to implement 21st Century Cures and what guidance you have been able to get from both OMB and the White House and which select user fee positions is the FDA hiring?

Dr. Woodcock. Well, I am not in a position to discuss that particularly, I can talk about what programmatic needs there will be. Clearly, the patient focused drug development is going to need different kind of scientists than we have traditionally had. We have had laboratory scientists who are looking in test tubes and doctors who are—we are going to need social scientists and other folks who can actually talk to people and get rigorous evidence about what their needs and preferences are and who can work on instruments, say, patient reported outcome measures and so forth. So that is one category that we don't necessarily have enough of.

In addition, on real-world evidence that is some different types of science that we will need to have people who can analyze that, big data, and so forth. And interesting, we have already had multiple outside parties approach us who are using real-world evidence in different ways and they want to collaborate with us and we are working with them, some of them in the Oncology Center of Excellence. So we will need data scientists of that sort.

And Breakthrough Therapy, which I know isn't Cures, but will need basically people who in specific disease areas particularly rare diseases. We also commit to integrate rare disease expertise within the review teams where there are rare diseases. We are seeing more and more rare diseases being treated.

So we have very focused needs in specific places for a specific kind of scientist, and I am sure that the Biologic Center with the rise in gene and cell therapy and that more or less explosion and also regenerative medicine, they are going to need specific types of scientific expertise.

Mr. Upton. Great. Well, thanks again for your work and we look forward to continuing the process as we get this thing done too. I yield back. Thank you, Mr. Chairman.

Mr. Guthrie. Thank you. The gentleman yields back and Mr. Schrader is recognized for 5 minutes.

Mr. Schrader. Thank you very much, Mr. Chairman, and thanks, Ms. Woodcock, for being here again. Very impressive results; I don't know if it is appropriate, but the graphs that are in your written testimony, I think, are pretty dramatic and you should share those with us when you come in and give your testimony. It would be pretty interesting, I think, for everyone to see that with the work of the committee and follow-through by FDA that the first drug approvals have dramatically increased and it is really pretty impressive. So make sure you show yourself to advantage when you become before us here.

I appreciated these comments on the Breakthrough Therapy Program with regard particularly to new and innovative drugs with unmet needs. We are finding that in the generic area that once again there are unmet needs despite the fact there may have been a product and there is either a sole source or no source alternative. Any thought of how the breakthrough process you are currently using on the brand name side might translate into the generic sphere of development?

Dr. Woodcock. Our analysis of the issues with generics is more that, you know, about ten percent of what we call reference drugs, the brand drugs, never get a generic filed to them. And so this seems to be a market phenomenon, competition is only attracted where people think they can make money by competing, and the small source products and so forth.

Now in the generic drug user fee program, the second one that we are proposing, the programmatic enhancements include a program to help with complex generics. And those are ones that actually people might not try to enter the market because it is hard, where, say, you are using an autoinjector or you are using a very complex molecule and so it might be hard.

So there, and we have agreed that we would set up a pre-program similar to kind of like the prescription drug user fee where before they send in the application we have meetings with them and we give them advice and we help them develop their products, so by the time they get the application in the door it actually could be approvable.

So that would help with those types of products, but the small——

Mr. Schrader. I guess where I was going—and that is very good and I think that is outstanding and hopefully a benefit to a lot of the companies out there. But I was going, say we are able to encourage a manufacturer to come to market through a variety of different means. We have a bill, Gus Bilirakis and I are trying to find what is the appropriate way to get and incentivize folks to come to market; make it worth their while as you put it.

But once they are there it would be nice if you used that break-through approach that has been so successful to also, you know, hasten things through. And I think to, and help us encourage them to come to market and be successful, if they knew that break- through approach was going to be applied that might incentivize things also.

Dr. Woodcock. Well, we would be happy to work with you. In medicine we have a saying: First do no harm. And sometimes there are unintended consequences and I think it would be worth discussing, because there is such a commercial hit that the innovators take when they get a generic competition on the market that any provisions that they can sue us about or send us citizen petitions or obstruct a process cause delays, and I believe that needs to be taken into account as you think about incentivizing.

Mr. Schrader. We are trying to do that. We have a REMS portion of our bill to try and make sure that it is being used appropriately for safety purposes and not block competition in the market. So we are trying to listen to you and your advice.

Dr. Woodcock. We would be happy to work with you in this.

Mr. Schrader. Second question on the biomarkers. I think that is a great idea because it takes as you said, many times it takes awhile to get these drugs to market and many of them do fail. And so a lot of the manufacturers want to have some idea if they are on the right track and you want to have some idea if they are on the right track, so early intervention and changing things would be appropriate.

Taking a blood pressure measurement or whatever the appropriate biomarker is, how do you follow through on that as the medication goes through the market, or a product goes through the market, to make sure that number one that the biomarker does turn out to be an accurate reflection of what the drug's ultimate outcome is, and then, once the drug is on the market, how do you go back and reassess the biomarkers to make sure they are actually meaningful indicators for you and for the companies?

Dr. Woodcock. We have a program known as Accelerated Approval. For some biomarkers such as blood pressure, their benefit is unequivocal and we don't need to keep proving over and over again that lowering blood pressure keeps you from getting strokes and so forth. We know that. But many other biomarkers are, quote, surrogate endpoints that we aren't a hundred percent sure that they are going to translate into benefit, and therefore we would give an accelerated approval it is called. That is kind of a misnomer, kind of misleading, but what that means is we are approving us based on the biomarker, but they have to do further studies. They are required to do further studies after approval to show that their drug actually causes clinical benefit.

So you get on the market earlier, that is the accelerated part, but you still have to deliver that proof.

Mr. Guthrie. Thanks. The gentleman's time has expired. I will recognize Mr. Lance for 5 minutes for questions.

Mr. Lance. Thank you very much, Mr. Chairman. It is always good to see you, Doctor. I am encouraged to see that the Rare Diseases Program staff will be integrated into review teams for rare disease development programs to provide unique expertise. Could you please speak to the relationship between PDUFA and 21st Century Cures as it relates to drug development tools such as real-world evidence, complex trial designs, and biomarkers, and the importance of getting the agreement to the President's desk by the end of July?

Dr. Woodcock. Certainly. Well, what was negotiated in PDUFA VI bolsters certain aspects of Cures with additional resources, and also would have specific timelines put in place and agreements. Some of those are slightly different, but we can reconcile them all kind of defaulting to whatever the earliest thing we agreed to is, we would do it then, all right.

Mr. Lance. Yes, Dr. Woodcock.

Dr. Woodcock. So, for example, real-world evidence, their guidance and so forth we would put out. 21st Century Cures has a broader qualification process, so it includes patient reported outcomes, clinical outcome assessment, as well as biomarkers, whereas the PDUFA agreement is about biomarkers. However, we are going to put up the same process for everything, the Cures process, which puts in place timelines and obligations on both the submitters and the agency. So we will put that across the board.

We expect, as you all know from our discussions, the biomarkers to be the most difficult part of this, and so the PDUFA gives, envisions more support for the biomarker qualification process.

Mr. Lance. Thank you. Dr. Woodcock, 21st Century Cures included a provision on combination products and that provision directs the agency to improve coordination between the Device and Drug Centers. Considering both Centers are involved in this process, should there be some coordination between the agreements?

Dr. Woodcock. Yes, and actually I believe there is. PDUFA VI provides some resources actually are envisioned for the Device Center, all right, to conduct these reviews. But I am pleased to say under the leadership of Dr. Rachel Sherman, who is deputy commissioner, we have made considerable progress already in combination products. We have put together a council, we have mapped the processes, we have improved the processes, we have developed standardized templates and so forth. So I think we have made a lot of progress already and that these efforts in Cures and in the user fee agreements will enhance that.

Mr. Lance. Do both Centers receive part of the user fee for combination products?

Dr. Woodcock. Yes.

Mr. Lance. Is that the way it works?

Dr. Woodcock. Yes.

Mr. Lance. And as I understand it, the goal in fiscal year 2019 is 50 percent, when the goal in fiscal year 2021 is 90 percent; is that accurate?

Dr. Woodcock. I believe so. That is how we typically structure these goals. If we haven't been keeping track the first year or so we try to find out what our baseline is. It may be 80 percent—we might hope so, OK—and then we ratchet it up after that.

Mr. Lance. Thank you, Dr. Woodcock.

And Mr. Chairman, I yield back 1 minute, 25 seconds.

Mr. Guthrie. The gentleman yields back and Mr. Cárdenas is recognized for 5 minutes for questions.

Mr. Cárdenas. OK. I will try to yield back a minute and 25 seconds or more to keep up with the program here. Thank you very much, Mr. Chairman, for holding this hearing.

Dr. Woodcock, what is the significance of September 2017 as far as your professional world goes?

Dr. Woodcock. If these various user fee programs are not reauthorized at that time, we must initiate processes to let go of the staff and wind down the program. There is money in all these agreements to do that. There is some money held back.

Mr. Cárdenas. Yes, money held back to wind it down——

Dr. Woodcock. That is all.

Mr. Cárdenas [continuing]. Which only expends over a few more months.

Dr. Woodcock. That is correct.

Mr. Cárdenas. Are many of the people that would be let go, per se, if we legislatively failed to do our job here, would that—you are talking about jobs, people who are specialists, or what kind of jobs are they?

Dr. Woodcock. Most of these are doctors and scientists. They are almost all at the Ph.D. or M.D. level. The physicians are generally some specialists, so we would have nephrologists or people who are specializing in medical imaging, and so hard to find people.

Mr. Cárdenas. Is it fair to say that getting so close to September 2017 creates kind of a little bit of nervousness amongst people who are trying to get their work done in such an environment?

Dr. Woodcock. Well, what we would expect is the productivity would slow down as we approach the brink, tremendously. This has happened once before where we approached it and we lose staff. Our people are heavily recruited into other jobs and they aren't paid as we have all discussed, they aren't paid as much as private sector. And so I would expect we would start to lose people very early who would leave before they got their notice.

Mr. Cárdenas. So to that point, if and when this, it seems to have happened before, the ramping up, once there is a restoration after the fact, isn't the ramping up many times harder than it was in the ramping down?

Dr. Woodcock. It is indeed. At least in the New Drugs Program where we need to hire physicians, the last time, and we didn't come to a reduction in force, we just came sort of close to that, it took more than a year for the New Drugs Program to recover its losses, and its recruitment rate was slowed down which it already is slow, because people have kind of lost faith in the viability of the program.

Mr. Cárdenas. And something such as a year of that revamping to just restore back to where it was, doesn't that cause a compounding effect potentially when it comes to the actual work being done going forward not only within the department but in the industry that happens to interact with you?

Dr. Woodcock. Well, we would have to prioritize very carefully what work would be done. Public safety would come first, obviously, and we would probably not be able to give all the advice that we would like to give or that people would like to have from us.

Mr. Cárdenas. So the stress is—I am interpreting this conversation as there would be stress involved in many ways actually expands beyond the department if in fact we weren't able to timely, in a timely fashion get this restored.

Dr. Woodcock. I believe that is very accurate.

Mr. Cárdenas. Do our job legislatively by the September '17 deadline.

Dr. Woodcock. Yes.

Mr. Cárdenas. OK. So briefly, Dr. Woodcock, when it comes to what we have done on 21st Century Cures, and your department is complicit in making sure that we do well with that. But at the same time, when it comes to biomarkers can you please discuss further how PDUFA VI will help with these efforts and what further biomarker development activities PDUFA VI will provide resources for?

Dr. Woodcock. Certainly. Both 21st Century Cures and the program envisioned in PDUFA VI both envision more effort going to biomarkers. 21st Century Cures sets up a structured program for what we call regulatory qualification, and what that means is new biomarkers, a different sort, we would tell people, the public, you can use this biomarker to make this decision about patients.

Now that can be a very heavy decision say if it is a safety biomarker. We are saying we are trusting human lives to the results of this biomarker. So there is a lot of scientific work that has to go in to make sure that biomarker is providing reliable information to make that decision.

And so what we are going to do, or are instructed to do under Cures and also under this PDUFA VI, is develop the evidence standards, OK. How much evidence, so everybody understands what kind of evidence you need in order to rely upon a new biomarker, and also then evaluate new nominated biomarkers through the Cures process that was set up against those evidence standards. So we have to do both of these, so we need the kind of scientists who are able to do that sort of work.

Mr. Guthrie. OK, thank you. The gentleman's time has expired.

Mr. Cárdenas. Thank you, Chairman.

Mr. Guthrie. Thank you. I now recognize Mr. Long for 5 minutes for questions.

Mr. Long. Thank you, Mr. Chairman, and thank you, Dr. Woodcock, for being here today. I would like to spend my time with you discussing a very vulnerable population, one that I personally focused on helping. Every year, nearly 200,000 newborns in the United States are admitted to neonatal intensive care units for treatment. Due to the numerous challenges and despite current pediatric incentives, the last new drug for this population was approved in 1999.

Last year my colleague on this committee Ben Ray Lujan and I introduced the Promoting Life-Saving New Therapies for Neonates Act and are working to introduce the bill this year. Our bill would create a new incentive model by providing a narrowly targeted, transferable exclusivity voucher to drug sponsors who successfully develop products for neonates.

Do you believe the current pediatric incentives have been successful in stimulating therapy development for newborns?

Dr. Woodcock. No, not particularly, I do not.

Mr. Long. Given the lack of development, can you identify the challenges that you see from a regulatory perspective at FDA as well as research and development challenges for the industry?

Dr. Woodcock. Well, I believe that we have taken steps recently along with the American Academy of Pediatrics and others, and our new head of pediatrics at FDA is a neonatologist. And together with her and others we have put together a network of NICUs, because part of the issue is the NICUs did not standardize their treatment protocols and so everyone had a different treatment protocol. So if we were going to ask a developer, a drug developer, to develop a drug in NICUs, every NICU director would want a different protocol.

So the first thing that had to be done was say what is the standard of care in the NICU, in the neonatal intensive care unit, and then you can say what are the biggest unmet medical needs for neonates, and then you can start talking about, OK, do we have a trial network or do we have some type of infrastructure that could actually evaluate a new therapy were it developed? And they are working on doing that internationally which is really good news. So I would be happy to update you on the progress on that.

Mr. Long. This is a tough population to test drugs on.

Dr. Woodcock. That is right.

Mr. LONG. Are there steps you believe we could take in the upcoming user fee process to help spur much needed development for this vulnerable patient population?

Dr. Woodcock. I don't know in user fee process. My belief is, and I have talked to the American Academy of Pediatrics about this, that the heads of neonatal intensive care units need to get their program together, decide what the standard of care is, decide what the unmet medical needs are, develop trial structures so they could test new drugs, and if they make—if you build it they will come, in my opinion. If you make a pathway clear that developers could use, then I believe they will develop products for neonates, sick neonates. And I believe it is needed.

Mr. Long. OK, thank you. And once again thank you for being here today taking your time to be with us.

And Mr. Chairman, I yield back.

Mr. Guthrie. The gentleman yields back. Ms. Matsui is recognized for 5 minutes for questions.

Ms. Matsui. Thank you, Mr. Chairman.

Thank you, Dr. Woodcock, for being here. It is wonderful to have you here. First of all, I want to mention that I am concerned with the President's budget proposal and how it might impact the work that this committee is doing to reauthorize these vital agreements that they have. And I don't think it would be wise to renegotiate the user fee agreements that FDA and the industry have worked so hard to reach, nor do I think it would be wise to impose drastic cuts to the agency's budget authority that would endanger the FDA's ability to collect these user fees. FDA performs many critical functions to keep our food and drugs safe and we cannot afford to compromise that.

Now I am particularly concerned about both the development and the final price of drugs for patients with rare diseases. These populations are often neglected and left with little or no treatments or cures. I want to ensure that we take advantage of our robust research efforts in this country for these rare disease patients.

I am pleased that there are many provisions in the negotiated PDUFA agreement that would make important advances for this rare disease community, particularly building on the effort to include the patient experience in drug development ensuring that staff at FDA who have expertise in rare disease are integrated across different centers.

Dr. Woodcock, can you elaborate on the provisions in PDUFA that would help patients with rare diseases?

Dr. Woodcock. Well, I believe the biggest help is actually going to be in the patient focused drug development. And why is that, because rare diseases often are so rare there are not any doctors who really know what happens to the people. And so what we are encouraging and we are seeing now is the patients are getting together and they are having their own patient focused drug development meetings.

They are collecting, and we have given some grants out to help with this, they are collecting natural history on their disease so people actually know what happens to someone with the rare disease. Often it is very disparate. Not everyone with that rare disease has the exact same course, so then it is even harder to study them.

So we are encouraging them to develop natural history so we can help with trial designs and then maybe even outcome measures, like what is the most burdensome part of the disease? What would they like ameliorated? So that then if a company comes along and wants to develop they have a pathway to develop. So that is all baked into these agreements in rigorous ways of collecting that information and helping patient groups so they can develop these things.

But also of course there is an agreement to integrate rare disease staff into review teams so that there is more, it is not all about blood pressure meds and gigantic trials and heart disease, OK, it is about people who have the very rare diseases pose different problems in development.

Ms. Matsui. Right. OK, can you talk more about the Break-through Therapy Program and what successes had it had and what additional resources help FDA with approval of innovative orphan therapies?

Dr. Woodcock. Well, we were completely surprised after the Breakthrough provisions were passed that we got so many applications, all right, and so it has been extremely successful in getting designations. We are only supposed to designate drugs that preliminary data, their early data they develop in the clinic shows it may be a game changer in the disease. It may change the disease; it isn't proven yet.

I can get back to you with the actual numbers, but we have designated hundreds of these to our surprise—we thought it would only be a handful—and we have approved many. And so this is great news for patients, because many times when we approve these they actually are a game changer for that disease.

Ms. Matsui. OK. That is wonderful. You testified that surrogate endpoints have been the basis for 60 percent of rare disease approvals. Can you explain surrogate endpoints in laymen's terms and why they are important for rare disease approvals?

Dr. Woodcock. Surrogate endpoints are something other than how a patient feels or functions or how long they live. So that is our gold standard for approval, it makes you feel better or makes you function better or it makes you live longer. But often diseases take a really long time, OK, to have their manifestations. And say for diseases where you are missing an enzyme—that is many rare diseases. So you are missing an enzyme and you start accumulating that substance inside your body instead of eliminating it.

Ms. Matsui. Right.

Dr. Woodcock. And we can give back these enzymes now, so sometimes we have accepted the fact that in vital organs that material goes away, all right. Well, that has to be really good news. It is not a hundred percent sure that doing that will reverse the symptoms of the disease, but it is pretty plausible, right? So often we give an accelerated approval like we were talking about saying, OK, we will get it on the market. All the patients can start taking this because is it removing this stuff from the body, but we want you to show with a registry or other that actually they are feeling better eventually, to make sure that is the truth.

Ms. Matsui. OK. Thank you very much, and I have gone past my time and I yield back.

Mr. Guthrie. Thank you. The time has expired, and we recognize Mr. Bilirakis for 5 minutes for questions.

Mr. Bilirakis. Thank you so much. I appreciate it, Mr. Chairman. And thank you, Dr. Woodcock, for coming today again.

Recently the FDA issued a request for comment on a proposed Office of Patient Affairs. Can you tell us what the goal of this office is, how it fits into the agency with its current patient related programs, and how this office would benefit patients?

Dr. Woodcock. The thought is that many patients don't understand the structure of FDA. FDA has long been divided into Centers, and if you are kind of inside Washington, you know you call the Biologic Center and you call the Drug Center. But what do you do if you don't know even who to call, right. So the thought is for medical products, not for foods or whatever, but for medical products, if people have questions about medical products there ought to be a little bit of a front-facing, patient-facing unit that can help people figure out who to ask the question. And so that is, I think, a lot of the rationale behind it.

Mr. Bilirakis. All right, thank you. Dr. Woodcock, in the 21st Century Cures Act we were able to pass reform language to modernize the Office of Combination Products. As you know, combination products are products on the market that have elements of a medical device and a drug, like inhalers and insulin injectors. Many patients need and rely on combination products, as you know.

While we worked on the 21st Century Cures, I asked FDA about innovation in the drug and device space as more and more innovative products may be combination products. At the time there were complaints from innovators about the slow and burdensome FDA process for approving combination products. One of your colleagues at FDA stated in an hearing, "That is a place that does require probably further discussion and whether or not there are changes to be thought about to make that intersection work better than it currently does."

Can you update us on what the FDA is doing on the drug side to implement the Cures language for combination products and what was agreed to in the user fee agreement?

Dr. Woodcock. Certainly. Well, what we are doing, the Cures product calls for work on this and the user fee program, the drug user fee program, actually provides resources for review of the device portion, OK, so that has been agreed to. But in advance of that we have set up a combination product council at the agency. We have mapped the different processes. We have revised them to make them more efficient. We are tracking them. We have standard forms and so forth, and I think everyone agrees that that is all going much better now.

So even in advance of implementing these we have gotten sort of the basics down about how to do these reviews more effectively given that we agree with you, this is the future of products. But the PDUFA program proposes that more resources be given to the Device Center to conduct these reviews of drug related, drug-led combination products of which many of these are.

Mr. Bilirakis. OK, very good. I yield back, Mr. Chairman. Thank you.

Mr. Guthrie. The gentleman yields back, and Ms. Eshoo is recognized for 5 minutes for questions.

Ms. Eshoo. Thank you, Mr. Chairman. Welcome, Dr. Woodcock.

Dr. Woodcock. Thank you.

Ms. Eshoo. It is always good to see you. Mr. Long is not here, but I wanted to say for the record that in FDASIA when we built that and passed it, I had language in that that required neonatologists being hired, and that was back in 2012. So I will talk to him later. I will be happy to work with him, but I think that that is important to set down for the record.

The PDUFA was enacted in 1992. I was running for Congress when that was put into place. And at that time drug review times were lagging and the FDA simply really couldn't keep up with the flood of new drug applications. So through these user fees paid by applicants it has given the FDA the resources it needed to hire and support more staff very specifically to move the applications forward.

I think the program overall has been successful at reducing review time backlogs, and even though the President criticized the FDA during his joint address to the Congress for, "having a slow and burdensome approval process," I think the facts really dispute that claim. And we are always looking to improve it, but it has been instrumental in promoting the improvements we have seen over the past 25 years.

Now I want to talk about two bills that I authored. I am very proud of them. One the BPCA, the Best Pharmaceuticals for Children Act; and the other, PREA, the Pediatric Research Equity Act. Both of these programs were permanently reauthorized in 2012, but I think today we need some improvements. We know that children are not just small adults; that drugs work differently in them than in adults and they have to be studied specifically for their use. That is why I authored both of these pieces of legislation. I think they have a track record of success, because more than 664 drug labels have been revised with important pediatric information as a result of the two bills.

So my question to you, Dr. Woodcock, is what is the implication of the orphan drug exemption in PREA on children's health? Are there examples of orphan drugs that would have benefited from a pediatric study but were not studied as a result of the orphan drug exemption in PREA?

Dr. Woodcock. I have to get back to you on specifics, are there any. In general, the orphan diseases, the rare diseases are sort of throughout life. Many of them start in childhood and so children are usually studied.

So much of the pediatric drug development problems were the fact that drugs were studied for adult diseases and there would be a few children who had them, relatively speaking, and they weren't ever studied, right, and it was used off-label in them, but in many of the rare diseases that rare disease starts in childhood and continues through.

But there may be some instances, and we can get back to you about where the rare disease predominates in adults. There are only a few children, and perhaps then the exemption means that those children may not be studied, but in talking to the rare disease and the orphan staff and the pediatric staff they don't believe this is a large problem.

Ms. Eshoo. Well, orphan drugs are, as you know they are currently exempt from PREA's——

Dr. Woodcock. Yes.

Ms. Eshoo [continuing]. Pediatric study requirements and that is why I am asking about it. Before the BPCA and PREA, the vast majority of drugs, more than 80 percent used in children were used off-label and without data on their safety or efficacy, and today that number has been reduced to approximately 50 percent, but that is still a lot. That is still a lot.

Why, if FDA has the authority to issue civil monetary penalties for other violations of the Food, Drug, and Cosmetic Act, including violations of post-marketing requirements, do you think that the FDA should be prohibited from using that authority to ensure compliance with PREA post-marketing requirements?

Dr. Woodcock. That is a legal question and we would be happy to work with you and get back to you on that.

Ms. Eshoo. But do you have any thoughts on it? You deal with legal all the time.

Dr. Woodcock. I do.

Ms. Eshoo. You live within a legal framework.

Dr. Woodcock. That is correct. The civil money penalties provisions and those provisions are apparently rather difficult to operate and implement, but so I would prefer getting back to you with the agencies.

Ms. Eshoo. Sure. That is fine. Thank you very much.

Thank you, Mr. Chairman.

Mr. Guthrie. Thank you. The lady yields back, and I now recognize Mrs. Blackburn for 5 minutes for asking questions.

Mrs. Blackburn. Thank you, Mr. Chairman.

Dr. Woodcock, you were so patient to come to us regularly, and we do appreciate it because we are so interested in making certain that things that are supposed to be done are tended to.

As Chairman Upton mentioned, 21st Century Cures, the implementation there, of course the Children Count Act which I had had that component, that is something that we are going to watch very closely and so we do appreciate the updates. We know it takes a lot of time to come up here, but we are very appreciative. I just want to quickly look at the abuse deterrent opioids and the components that are there. March 2016, you did the draft guidance. When is there going to be the final guidance on that? What is the expectation?

And then I want to know, I know we have touched around the edges on this, but talk a little bit about the actions that can and should be taken from you all to advance the abuse deterrent opioids and to get these into the marketplace, just a little bit there. And that is really my only two questions.

Dr. Woodcock. Certainly. Well, as far as the guidance, it is very difficult ever to give a firm date certain when a final is going to come out.

Mrs. Blackburn. Just an expectation or timeline.

Dr. Woodcock. Well, let me just assure you that we are putting great effort into this, because really what we need to do, we think, is incentivize innovator development of various abuse deterrent formulations. The current ones, as we have already discussed, are kind of version 1.0 and surely we can do better, right. And so there has to be probably some incentives there.

And then generics, we need a pathway so that the generics understand what they would have to do to show that they source exactly the same as the innovator, because uptake of these abuse deterrent formulations is lower because there are a lot of old opioids on the market that are very inexpensive that are not abuse deterrent.

And that is often for health systems the preferred opioid to use to save money, so we need a progression of incentives and also a clear pathway. But the innovation needs to go from the innovators, the people who are out there trying to figure out better ways to deter abuse.

Mrs. Blackburn. Right, but are we talking 6 months, a year? I mean, when do you think there will be a final decision——

Dr. Woodcock. A final guidance for the generic?

Mrs. Blackburn. Yes.

Dr. Woodcock. I would hope within 6 months, I certainly would.

Mrs. Blackburn. That is great. And then if you will speak just a little bit toward what further the FDA can do to spur the abuse deterrent opioids.

Dr. Woodcock. Sure. There are many things we are trying to do, one of them though is trying to incentivize development of drugs, new drugs that don't have these abuse liabilities to treat pain, and we have approved a number of them. They are often for specific conditions.

For example, we approved one for neuropathic pain and that is now being used by the neurologist, those drugs, instead of opioids because opioids aren't very good for neuropathic pain. So that cuts out one category of people who are getting these opioids.

So we want to stimulate and we have been working on this for years with the outside world, scientific world, trying to stimulate the development of drugs that aren't opioids that don't have these abuse liabilities, because people are going to continue prescribing opioids for people in pain unless they have something else to offer. So also we have workshops and we work on abuse deterrent formulations to try and stimulate and work with innovators on new ways to deter abuse.

Mr. Griffith. The gentlelady yields back. Mr. Butterfield is recognized for 5 minutes for questions.

Mr. Butterfield. Thank you very much, Mr. Chairman.

Let me just begin by thanking you and Dr. Woodcock, for coming back. You have been at that table many times and thank you so very much. Chairman Burgess, who is not here today, but I want to thank him for holding this hearing on the Prescription Drug User Fee Agreement reauthorization.

Since I came to Congress some 12 years ago back in '04, Congress has come together under the leadership of both Democrats and Republicans to pass this important bipartisan legislation. Just last year we passed the 21st Century Cures Act that this committee drafted and passed unanimously to help boost the resources of the Food and Drug Administration and encourage the development of new treatments.

For my constituents in North Carolina, developing new treatments can literally make the difference between life and death. Health outcomes for many in the communities that I represent are deeply concerning. Many of my constituents are African American citizens. By most measurable health statistics, outcomes for African Americans lag far behind. Supporting the reauthorization of PDUFA is important to finding new treatments to help reduce health disparities for my constituents and indeed Americans all across the country.

Through additional resources made possible by PDUFA V, the FDA has been able to work with industry to make available new treatments for rare diseases through the Breakthrough Therapy Program. Through

November of last year, FDA has granted, I am told, 165 breakthrough therapy requests. This includes treatment in many areas that disproportionately impact my constituents and African Americans throughout the country.

Breakthrough designations have been granted for diseases like HIV and hepatitis C, and colorectal cancer, all of which impact minorities at high rates. PDUFA VI has the potential to make advancements in areas from breakthrough therapies and real-world evidence to clinical trials and biomarkers. The additional resources made possible through the proposed new fee structure can help FDA build the workforce needed to complete these new tasks.

However, this administration's executive actions and proposed budget do not seem to understand the importance of FDA's mission to help patients and improve public health. The impact of a hiring freeze on the FDA implemented by the Trump administration is still unclear. Also the administration's budget proposal fails to understand the good-faith effort that has been put forth by the FDA and by industry and patient advocacy groups all working together. Now is the time to come together to support the FDA. Our constituents are counting on us, my colleagues, to work together in this space.

Dr. Woodcock, I am excited by the innovations occurring in cancer drug development as cancer drugs are now being developed by molecular target. By identifying the drivers of the cancers, these new molecularly targeted drugs are achieving great new strides in treatment and providing greater health to cancer patients. These targeted drugs are often effective for many types of cancers.

Question, are innovative new cancer treatments for adults also tested for children with the same targets as adult cancers?

Dr. Woodcock. Not generally. The paradigm is changing and typically over time treatments for cancer as well as other disorders have been according to disease. So in cancer it is what we call histology, which basically means the organ that the cancer originated in. That is why we call it colon cancer or we call it whatever cancer, lung cancer, right.

But these molecular alterations may go across diseases and it may be only a small subset of each of these cancers are driven by the same molecular alteration. That isn't something that has really been looked at very closely in children. It may be that there are rare mutations in children that are the similar as the mutation in adult for these molecular targeted therapies.

Mr. Butterfield. OK. Also my colleague Representative McCaul of Texas and I introduced the RACE for Children Act, H.R. 1231, to promote the discovery of new cures for children with cancer. First, the RACE for Children Act would provide that a drug company will provide a pediatric study plan of a drug pursuant to the Pediatric Research Equity Act if the drug is, ''intended for the treatment of an adult cancer and is directed at a molecular target considered to be germane to the growth and progression of such pediatric cancer."

Do you believe this provision would create greater access to novel cancer drugs for pediatric cancer research?

Dr. Woodcock. I am not able to comment on that at this time, but we would be happy to work with you on this.

Mr. Butterfield. All right. We are deep into this and we would like all the help we can get. Secondly, the RACE for Children Act would end the—I am over, yes. I yield back.

Mr. Guthrie. I yield back. Thank you for yielding back. I see no questions on the majority side. Mr. Sarbanes, you are recognized for 5 minutes for questions.

Mr. Sarbanes. Thank you, Mr. Chairman.

Thank you, Dr. Woodcock, for joining us. I have been here 10 years, I think on four or five different committees. You are my all-time favorite witness. I just want you to know that. Because you are so professional in your presentations, so knowledgeable, and you play things straight, so I appreciate your being here.

I am fascinated by this idea of including, incorporating real-world evidence in regulatory decision making. I mean the implications of it are kind of humorous because it suggests that up until now there hasn't been real-world evidence in the process, but I certainly understand what it is meant to convey.

And I was wondering if you would just talk a little bit about that topic. And obviously the agency is going to have to come up with, and I know you are in the process of doing this, a kind of formal process for identifying what qualifies as real-world evidence and then how it gets gathered and then how it gets translated back to the agency, how much weight is given to it as part of the overall analysis that is done by the staff there at the FDA. So if you could maybe just talk about that a little bit more that would be helpful.

Dr. Woodcock. Certainly. Well, FDA runs actually one of the largest real-world evidence gathering operations that is around in the health area, which is our Sentinel System, which is for drug safety and was mandated by Congress. And there we have 193 million different people's claims data that we can access, all right, anonymously, and we use that for drug safety analysis.

And the Congress told us that that should be used first rather than requiring companies perhaps to do specific observational studies. And recently, as we have institutionalized this system there are four programs where we are able to do something in Sentinel and not require additional outside studies, but that is safety.

Now on the effectiveness side, obviously you would only collect real-world data if the drug were on the market, OK, because before a drug gets on the market data is collected into clinical trials, it is not just collected into doctor's offices. So that would be after a drug is marketed can we collect patient experience data to perhaps broaden the indication or add new indications or whatever.

Mr. Sarbanes. Can you comment on how sort of off-label use relates to that?

Dr. Woodcock. Well, it does relate to it, because often, for example, let's take these oncology drugs and these targeted drugs. So they target a specific target. We may approve it for a number of tumors, but then there may be somebody who comes in and they have a rare tumor or a tumor that this is an unusual type and they have that mutation. So the physician may treat them with the targeted agent and that would be considered off-label use although it is completely rational, right.

So what we are working with a large number of outside parties who are gathering this information up in different ways and then they want to collect that experience of the patients, those rare patients, and then perhaps if they responded and we can document that then maybe we can add that to the label and say if you have a rare patient like this come in they should be treated with this targeted therapy too. So that is an example.

There also are registries, and some people consider those real-world evidence and some don't. But we are trying to put registries together, get that registry information, make sure it is——

Mr. Sarbanes. Just on that point again intrigued me. What would make certain people consider a registry real-world evidence and other people not consider it real-world evidence?

Dr. Woodcock. Yes. Well, some people are sort of purists and they consider real-world evidence only collected like in the course of ordinary medical care and of stock, OK. Other people consider it evidence that is collected during the course of treatment even if you add a few bells and whistles. So we really don't care. This is evidence outside of standard clinical trials, so let's figure out for all of it what can we do to gather more information about performance of drugs outside of your traditional clinical trial.

Mr. Sarbanes. Would you imagine that at the end of this process adding this to your portfolio, if you want to call it that, that there would be maybe some kind of advisory council or group that the FDA would bring into the process of identifying real-world evidence? I mean, what kind of structures do you think we might see, or is it premature to——

Dr. Woodcock. I think what you would see is a series of policy sort of guidances or pronouncements by the FDA as we are able to broaden our uses of and examples of how we have used it. And in some of those cases we may take it to a specific advisory committee, say we think we should add these, say, tumors to the label because here is the real-world experience and it looks like these people respond and they would never get in a clinical trial because they are rare or whatever.

So that I think is the kind of accumulating information. We can't just have people sort of think great thoughts absent examples of what can be done.

Mr. Sarbanes. Right, thanks very much. I yield back.

Mr. Guthrie. Yes, thanks, time has expired. And seeing no other members here to ask questions—well, thank you, Dr. Woodcock, for being here. I concur it is always great to have you here and you always do a good job. I appreciate it.

Dr. Woodcock. Thank you.

Mr. Guthrie. We will now transition to our second panel.

Thank you. We want to thank all of the witnesses for being here today and taking the time to testify before the subcommittee. As a reminder, each witness will have the opportunity to give an opening statement followed by a round of questions for members.

Our second panel of witnesses includes Mr. Jeff Allen, President and CEO, Friends of Cancer Research; Ms. Kay Holcombe, Senior Vice President of Science Policy, Biotechnology Industry Organization; and Dr. Anne Pritchett, Vice President of Policy and Research, Pharmaceutical Research and Manufacturers of America.

We appreciate you all being here, and we will begin the panel with Mr. Allen, and you are now recognized for 5 minutes for an opening statement.

Statements Of Jeff Allen, Phd, President And Ceo, Friends Of Cancer Research; Kay Holcombe, Senior Vice President Of Science Policy, Biotechnology Industry Organization; And, Anne Pritchett, Phd, Vice President Of Policy And Research, Pharmaceutical Research And Manufacturers Of America

STATEMENT OF JEFF ALLEN

Mr. Allen. Good morning, Vice Chairman Guthrie, Ranking Member Green, and members of the subcommittee. It is an honor to be here today to provide the perspective of Friends of Cancer Research. The current pace of scientific discovery represents an unparalleled opportunity to improve human health. The critical component to this is an FDA that is highly responsive to public health needs and able to evolve with cutting edge science.

Prior to the initial user fee authorization in 1992, patients in other parts of the world were gaining access to new medicines more readily than Americans with only about ten percent of new treatments reaching U.S. patients first. Today that paradigm has been reversed. Funds through the PDUFA mechanism have allowed the FDA to make the review process more predictable, efficient, and accessible. In fact, our data indicates that for new cancer drugs approved by both the FDA and the European counterpart, 97 percent were available in the United States first. Furthermore, the FDA approved them on average nearly 6 months faster.

This sixth authorization of the user fee agreement comes at a critical time for the agency and for patients. It will support numerous initiatives, a couple of which I would like to mention today. PDUFA VI advances the role of patients and their experiences. PDUFA V, in the 21st Century Cures Act, provided important steps to incorporate the patient perspective in drug development.

The PDUFA VI agreement will further assist organizations, researchers, in collecting patient experience data, create channels for providing such data to the FDA, and it will help develop methods for analyzing it. PDUFA VI supports the Breakthrough Therapy Designation. This designation to expedite the development of highly promising new drugs has been rapidly implemented. To date, 170 designations have been granted leading to 79 approvals.

Upon examining the pre-market development time of new cancer drugs, we found that it was over 2 years shorter for breakthrough designated drugs than for those without the designation. PDUFA VI will provide resources necessary for continued success. PDUFA VI promotes qualification and use of drug development tools that can help identify patients for which a drug is likely to work, offer early indicators of toxicity to help improve patient safety, and in some cases indicate that a drug will have long term benefit. The agreement will help create a process in which new tools can be accurately assessed and ensure their appropriate use.

PDUFA VI enhances the use of real-world evidence. Once a drug reaches real-world populations there may be unanswered questions about its effects, particularly in patients not represented in clinical trials. The collection of real-world evidence allows for a greater understanding of drugs currently in use. By allocating user fee funding toward these programs, the FDA and other stakeholders will be able to identify limitations and explore different opportunities for the use of data collected from post-market experience.

To that end, FDA approved labels should be a vitally important source of information to guide the safe and effective use of prescription drugs. However, in some instances, such as drugs that have gone off patent, labels may have become outdated and no longer reflect optimal use. This is illustrated by extensive discrepancies between FDA approved labels and widely accepted practice guidelines.

The FDA could play a greater role in evaluating the relevant data to update the product label as appropriate and adjudicate between the uses backed by strong evidence and those backed by less persuasive information. This would establish a high standard for post-market evidence and make the product labels more useful. For the programs of this proposed user fee agreement to succeed, the full budget of the FDA must be robust and the capacity of which the agency can maintain and hire the best scientific minds must be unencumbered.

Despite opportunities afforded by PDUFA VI, the passage of the 21st Century Cures Act, and the enormous contributions of this committee, I would be remiss to state that the FDA and the people who rely on it are optimally positioned at present. The proposed cuts to biomedical research will put the brakes on the engines of discovery and jeopardize the development of new medicines for patients. Holding the FDA budget authority at stagnant levels prevents progress on agency functions that are not covered by user fees.

Among the challenges that have been exacerbated in the current environment is the implementation of the FDA Oncology Center for Excellence, an innovative approach and a new model for collaboration. The potential of a detrimental budget and the presence of the current hiring freeze put the OCE and so many other transformational opportunities at significant risk. For the people who currently depend on safe and effective medicines, for those who are holding strong for the breakthroughs to come, and for every future patient, there isn't time to waste. We urge Congress to swiftly pass the sixth reauthorization of PDUFA. Thank you.

[The prepared statement of Jeff Allen follows:]

FRIENDS of CANCER RESEARCH

Examining FDA's Prescription Drug User Fee Program

Testimony Before Committee on Energy and Commerce Subcommittee on Health United States House of Representatives

Jeff Allen, PhD

President & CEO

Friends of Cancer Research

March 22, 2017

Examining FDA's Prescription Drug User Fee Program

Testimony of Jeff Allen, PhD, President & CEO, Friends of Cancer Research

Few in biomedical science can recall a time of greater scientific progress. Hardly a day goes by without reports of a new medical breakthrough, a new partnership to drive discovery forward, or a new milestone toward addressing a previously untreatable disease. This pace of scientific discovery represents an unparalleled opportunity to improve human health. While it offers great hope for the future, progress has not been universal, and significant challenges remain. In the field of oncology, certain types of cancer are no longer the deadly diseases they once were, but instead are much like chronic conditions that can be effectively managed for a lifetime. But other types of cancer have not seen a new treatment for decades, if at all, leaving some to wonder if they will ever reap the benefits of progress.

The drugs and biologics being developed today to treat many diseases are far more effective than their predecessors, but they're also more complex. Even for some of the most notable new advancements benefit only a subset of patients. This additional complexity adds to the process of developing a new medicines, which already reportedly takes upwards of 12 years and costs over $1 billion.[2] But together we have the opportunity to support breakthrough science, design systems that can surmount new challenges, and pave the way for new discoveries to reach the people who need them most. I, and millions of people across this country, hope that the work of this committee will be a catalyst to accelerate getting the right medicines to the right patients at the right time.

A critical component to achieving this goal is a well-resourced, accessible, and scientifically-oriented Food & Drug Administration (FDA). The FDA continues to be an agency that is highly responsive to public health needs and evolves with cutting edge science. It is able do so, in part, because of the Prescription Drug User Fee Act (PDUFA).

THE PRESCRIPTION DRUG USER FEE ACT

PDUFA was first passed in 1992 to alleviate a backlog of new drug applications. Prior to the initial user- fee authorizations, patients in other parts of the world were gaining access to new medicines more readily than Americans, with only about 10% of new treatments reaching U.S. patients first.[3] Today, that paradigm has largely been reversed. Funds provided though the PDUFA mechanism have allowed the FDA to clear the backlog

---

[2] Adams, C. P. and Brantner, V. V. Health Economics, 19 (2010), 130–141. doi: 10.1002/hec.1454

[3] Hearing of the Committee on Health, Education, Labor, and Pensions, US Senate: FDA User Fee Agreements: Strengthening FDA and the Medical Products Industry for the Benefit of Patients. 112th Congress. March 29, 2012. https://www.gpo.gov/fdsys/pkg/CHRG-112shrg90814/html/CHRG-112shrg90814.htm Accesses 3.17.17

of applications and have made the review process more predictable, efficient, and accessible. As a result, patients in this country have gained timely access to new medicines. In fact, in a study that we first published in Health Affairs,[4] we examined the review times for new oncology drugs by the FDA and its European counterpart, the European Medicines Agency (EMA). Between the years 2003 and 2016, 73 new cancer drugs were approved by both the FDA and EMA. Of those drugs, 97% (71 of 73) were available in the U.S. before Europe. Furthermore, the FDA approved new cancer drugs on average nearly 6 months faster than the EMA (Figure 1). Other research groups have also demonstrated that FDA regularly approves products faster than other global regulatory agencies and that this is the case for all drug reviews, not just for oncology drugs.[5]

The initial PDUFA authorizations were an indisputable success in speeding FDA review times and injecting greater predictability into the way drugs are approved by the agency. However, their initial impact was limited to the period after a new drug application was submitted to the FDA, leaving the much lengthier development process that precedes FDA review unaddressed. But the period in which the FDA reviews a new drug application accounts for only a fraction of the time that it frequently takes to develop a new medicine. Since then, however, the FDA has become increasingly involved at earlier stages of the development process. As such, the FDA has played an increasingly important and active role in reviewing interim results from earlier stage studies, and has provided feedback on research study designs through a variety of meetings with clinical study sponsors. The FDA has also played an increasingly active and valuable role in providing regulatory perspectives and participating in scientific discussions outside of activities related to a specific product application.

---

[4] Roberts S, Allen J, and Sigal E. *Despite Criticism Of The FDA Review Process, New Cancer Drugs Reach Patients Sooner In The United States Than In Europe.* Health Aff July 2011 vol. 30 no. 71375-1381: http://content.healthaffairs.org/content/30/7/1375.full.html Accessed 3.17.17

[5] Downing NS, Aminawung JA, Shah ND, Braunstein JB, M.D., Krumholz HM, Ross JS. *Regulatory Review of Novel Therapeutics — Comparison of Three Regulatory Agencies.* N Engl J Med 2012; 366:2284-2293: http://www.nejm.org/doi/full/10.1056/NEJMsa120022 3#t=article Accessed 3.17.17

Over time, the FDA's more active role in product development has led to expansions to the agreements between the FDA and the drug manufacturers that supply the user fees. Recent user fee agreements have allowed funds to be applied to activities that are beyond the primary application review functions, such as programs to advance the science that serves as the basis for new product development. In addition to funding core product review and personnel, the sixth authorization of the user fee agreement will support key projects that ensure the FDA can conduct critical scientific programing, participate in public workshops, and develop guidance for its employees and external stakeholders regarding cutting-edge science and new strategies for drug development and regulation.

Drugs Approved by FDA and EMA **n = 73**		
	FDA	**EMA**
Median Review Time (in days)	183	356
# Drugs reviewed w/in 6 months	36 (49%)	1 (1%)
# Drugs reviewed w/in 1 year	70 (96%)	45 (62%)

Figure 1. Comparison of FDA and EMA Review of New Oncology Drugs (2003-2016).

HIGHLIGHTS OF THE PDUFA IV AGREEMENT

PDUFA VI Advances the Role of Patients and Their Experiences

As part of the PDUFA V programs, the FDA began to build a robust Patient Focused Drug Development program. This included quarterly public meetings with patients, caregivers, advocates, and FDA personnel. Each meeting focused on a specific disease and was designed to gain insights directly from people who experience that condition on how it impacts their daily lives. The 21st Century Cures Act takes important steps to operationalize this type of feedback. It begins to set up processes to assist organizations and researchers in collecting patient-experience data, creates channels for providing such data to the FDA, and it will help develop methods for analyzing it.[6] The PDUFA VI agreement further builds on these programs and sets the course for further incorporation of the patient voice in drug development. Under the agreement, user fees will be used to hold public workshops, develop guidance documents, strengthen internal capacity, and establish new methods for clinical outcomes assessments and patient reported outcome measures.

PDUFA VI Supports the Continued Success of the Breakthrough Therapy Designation

In 2012, the FDA Safety and Innovation Act (FDASIA), which contained the reauthorization of PDUFA V, established the Breakthrough Therapy Designation. This designation may be given to a drug intended to treat a serious illness for which preliminary clinical evidence indicates a substantial improvement over any existing intervention.[7] This designation was rapidly implemented into drug development programs, and to date, 170 Breakthrough Therapy Designations have been granted, leading to 79 indications approved by FDA using this process (Figure 2).

When the Breakthrough Therapy Designation is granted by the FDA, an intense collaboration is initiated between the agency and the sponsor to expedite the development of the drug. This process results in near real-time interactions between the FDA and sponsors, the involvement of senior leadership at the FDA, use of cross disciplinary project teams for optimal coordination of different application components, and consideration of different study designs that can minimize the number of patients exposed to inferior agents throughout clinical testing. While these process enhancements can add efficiencies to the development process of drugs that demonstrate extraordinary clinical activity, they are also resource intensive. As indicated in Figure 2 by the more than 500 requests for Breakthrough Therapy Designation received since FDASIA established the

---

[6] PL 114-255. The 21st Century Cures Act. Title III Subtitle A Patient Focused Drug Development

[7] PL 112-144. FDASIA Sec. 902 Breakthrough Therapies.

designation in 2012, it is a widely-used program that continues to demand a heavy workload from the FDA.

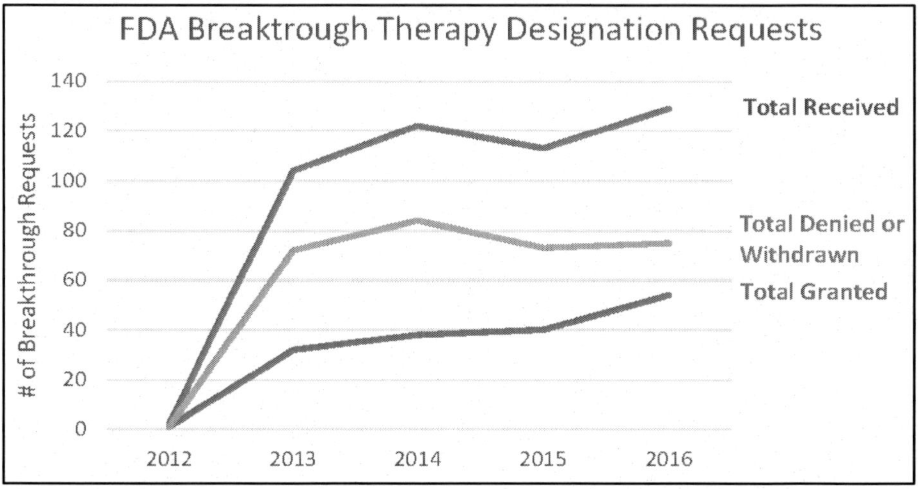

Year	Total Received	Total Granted	Total Denied	Total Withdrawn
2012	2	1	1	0
2013	104	32	62	10
2014	122	38	70	14
2015	113	40	52	21
2016	129	54	62	13
2017	35	5	8	0
Total	**505**	**170**	**255**	**58**

Data source: US Food and Drug Administration

Figure 2. Breakthrough Therapy Designation Use 2012-2016.

In a recent analysis to explore the impact of the designation for new oncology products, we found that breakthrough-designated cancer drugs were reviewed in an average timeframe 3 months shorter than for those without the designation. While review times are important, the key goal of the Breakthrough Therapy Designation is to expedite drug development. It does so by acknowledging that new drugs demonstrating transformative potential early in their clinical testing may be permitted to employ novel approaches to demonstrate the safety and efficacy required for approval. Upon examining the pre-market development time of new cancer drugs, calculated as the number of years from submission of an investigational new drug (IND) application to submission of a new drug application (NDA) or biologics license application (BLA), we found that development time was 2.2 years shorter for approved breakthrough-designated drugs than for those without the designation.[8] While this may be attributed in part to differences in natural disease trajectory of different cancers, the observed difference in development times provides preliminary evidence for the positive impact of the Breakthrough Therapy Designation and the collaboration it spurs. It is important to note that the Breakthrough Therapy Designation has been applied in a variety of different disease settings (Figure 3), with under half of publicly disclosed designations going to products that treat forms of cancer.

The PDUFA VI agreement will provide critical resources to allow the successful Breakthrough Therapy Designation to continue to facilitate rapid access to highly promising new medicines for patients suffering from serious diseases.

PDUFA VI Promotes Qualification and Use of Drug Development Tools

Developing new drugs is an incredibly risky process. The probability of an experimental drug compound progressing from Phase 1 trials to FDA approval was recently estimated to be 9.6% for all drug categories and 5.1% in oncology.[9] A major driver of this low success rate is the uncertainty drug developers face when testing a new drug. It takes time and careful study to identify whether the patients selected for a clinical study are most likely to benefit from an experimental therapy and to determine how they respond to treatment. Questions such as: "Is a patient

---

[8] Shea M, et al. *Impact of breakthrough therapy designation on cancer drug development.* Nat Rev Drug Dis. Vol. 15 p. 152. March 2016.

[9] Clinical Development Success Rates 2006-2015. BIO, Biomedtracker, Amplion: 2016. Accessed at: https://www.bio.org/sites/default/files/Clinical%20Development%20Success%20Rates%202006-2015%20-%20BIO,%20Biomedtracker,%20Amplion%202016.pdf Accessed 3.19.17

likely to develop side effects?" and "How far has the disease progressed?" and "Does a potential treatment target the correct disease pathway?" are routinely asked by drug developers and can be addressed efficiently through the use of biomarkers and other drug development tools.[10] They help researchers answer these questions by providing rapid, reliable information on key metrics including drug safety, pharmacodynamics and drug response.

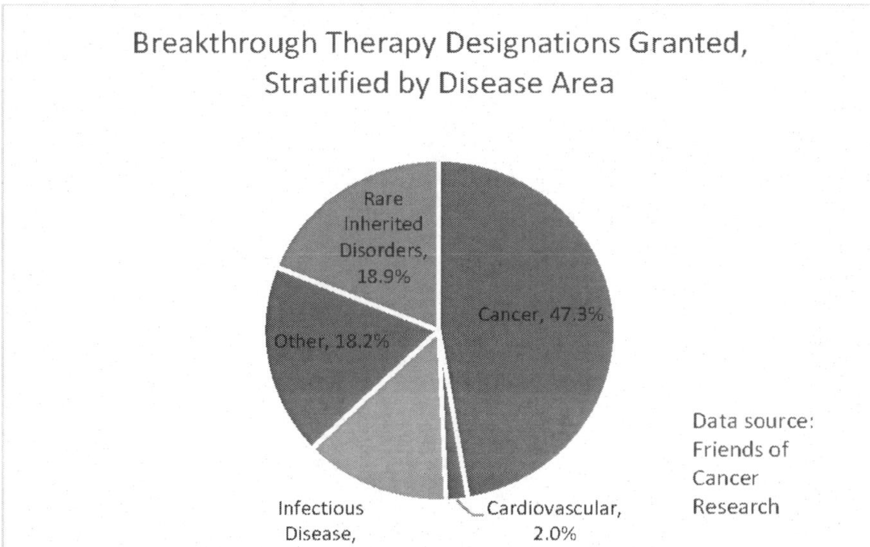

Figure 3. Breakthrough Designations by Disease.

The FDA has a program to "qualify" certain biomarkers and other drug-development tools, which provides drug developers with the assurance that the methods they use have been scientifically vetted. This has the potential to rapidly speed the pace of drug development and prevent waste created by the case-by-case approach to biomarker qualification that the FDA has adopted in the past.[11]

---

[10] Amur S, LaVange L, Zineh I, Buckman-Garner S, Woodcock J. Biomarker Qualification: Toward a Multiple Stakeholder Framework for Biomarker Development, Regulatory Acceptance, and Utilization. *Clinical Pharmacology & Therapeutics*. Volume 98 Number 1: July 2015.

[11] Ibid.

The present PDUFA reauthorization package contains important provisions to enhance the biomarker qualification process. It instructs the FDA to publish two draft guidance documents on standards and taxonomy for biomarker qualification, as well as to convene a public workshop to engage the public on these topics.

By facilitating the development of new markers that can serve as intermediate indicators of safety or efficacy, the clinical testing process is improved. The use of validated biomarkers can help identify patients for which a drug is likely to work, offer early indicators of toxicity that help improve patient safety, and in some cases indicate that a drug will have a longer term benefit and allow for earlier access to promising new drugs. The resources provided in the PDUFA VI agreement will help create a process in which new biomarkers and other drug development tools can be accurately assessed and ensure their appropriate use.

PDUFA VI Enhances the Use of Real-World Evidence in Regulatory Decision-Making

Clinical trials are typically conducted in highly controlled populations to maximize the probability of success. However, once a drug reaches real-world populations, there may be unanswered questions about a drug's effect in patients with characteristics not represented in clinical trials. The collection of real-world evidence (RWE) allows for a greater understanding of drugs currently in use. Real-world evidence is gathered by processing data from electronic medical records (EMRs) and tracking patient outcomes over time. This type of evidence has the potential to supplement the knowledge gained from pre-market studies and can aid in regulatory decision-making. Under PDUFA VI, the FDA will engage patients, industry and academia to better understand how RWE can be collected and used to support high-quality evidence generation and regulatory decision-making.

By allocating user-fee funding toward these programs, the FDA and other stakeholders will be able to identify limitations and explore different opportunities for the use of data collected from post-market experience with a drug.

FOR ADDITIONAL CONSIDERATION

Effectively Communicating Scientific Advances

Rapid advancement in science and technology allows our understanding of new and current drugs continues to grow. In the years following FDA approval, new data about drug safety and efficacy emerges rapidly through post-market clinical studies and real-world experience captured in day-to-day medical practice. While new safety information is readily incorporated into drug labeling, new information about drug efficacy is often not submitted to FDA for labeling updates. Despite its absence on approved labeling, new information is quickly synthesized by clinical guideline developers, which is then used to inform clinical practice. This drives the high rate of off-label prescribing, which has become commonplace; indeed between one half and three quarters of all oncology prescribing is done off label.[12] That off-label use is based on varying levels of supportive evidence. One study found that 27% of off-label uses were backed by strong evidence, with the remaining uses lacking strong scientific support.[13]

After reviewing collections of drug-related information published by clinical-guideline developers, called compendia, we found additional evidence of off-label use. When we compared drug compendia to existing FDA drug labels, we found that compendia recommended additional uses beyond the scope of those described in product labels for 79% of oncology

---

[12] Mullins CD, Montgomery R, Abernethy AP, Hussain A, Pearson SD, Tunis S; American Society of Clinical Oncology. Recommendations for clinical trials of off-label drugs used to treat advanced-stage cancer. J Clin Oncol. 2012 Feb 20;30(6):661-6.

[13] Radley D, Finkelstein S, Stafford R. Off-label Prescribing Among Office-Based Physicians. Arch Intern Med. 2006 May 8;166(9):1021-6.

drugs. Of the additional uses recommended by compendia, 91% were recommended by uniform consensus among the physicians developing the guidelines and recognized as acceptable uses by the four largest private insurers.

The variance between FDA labels and drug compendia indicates that there is a significant opportunity to improve how emerging scientific evidence can be incorporated into product labels. Currently, sponsors can submit a supplemental new drug application to modify a product label with additional efficacy claims. However, there may be instances when the efficacy profile of a drug has evolved but no supplemental application to the label was ever submitted. This typically happens when incentives to submit additional information are limited, such as when a drug has gone off patent and faces generic competition, or when a drug is no longer actively marketed.

Because PDUFA VI tasks the FDA and other stakeholders with exploring uses of post-market evidence, we believe that such information needs to be scientifically rigorous to appropriately inform patient and practitioner decisions. When post-market data presents compelling evidence for a new use of an approved product, the FDA could play a greater role in evaluating the relevant data to update the product label, as appropriate. This would allow independent experts at FDA to adjudicate between uses backed by strong evidence and those backed by less persuasive evidence, and to establish a standard by which post-market evidence should be evaluated.

Restoring the relevance of FDA-approved labels is an important public health goal. While other high quality sources of clinical prescribing information exist, FDA labels remain the sole source of information carrying the weight of a scientific agency with decades of experience reviewing drug efficacy data. Ensuring that processes are in place to modify outdated product labels can help ensure that use of the product is supported by the highest quality of evidence possible, and that patients and physicians can have confidence in supplemental uses of approved drugs.

CURRENT CHALLENGES TO THE FDA

Despite opportunities afforded by PDUFA VI, the passage of the 21st Century Cures Act, and the enormous contributions of this committee, I would be remiss to state that the FDA and the people who rely on it are optimally positioned at present. Even so, proposed cuts to biomedical research will put the brakes on the engine of discovery, abandon progress on new tools to enhance product evaluation, impede opportunities for new businesses in the biotech sector, and most perilously, jeopardize the development of new medicines for patients desperate for progress. Holding the FDA budget authority at stagnant levels prevents progress on agency functions that are not applicable to user fees. These include critical functions of the agency such as drug-safety surveillance programs, oversight of drug compounding facilities, review of product advertising material, oversight of over-the-counter medicines, and conduct of scientific programing. Compounded with the constraints of the federal hiring freeze, the FDA will be hamstrung. The ramifications will be felt for years to come.

Among the challenges that have been exacerbated in the current environment is the implementation of the FDA Oncology Center of Excellence (OCE). The 21st Century Cures Act included a directive for the agency to establish an initiative to coordinate activities within the three current medical product centers around one or more major disease areas.[14] To begin this work, the FDA established the OCE in recognition that cancer has evolved to require multimodal technologies for optimal management. For example, drugs are being developed with increased frequency to treat cancer using genetic information to guide their use. This can involve review divisions of CDER for the drug product, or CBER in instances of cell-based gene therapy or vaccines, and CDRH for a diagnostic. Housing these functions and expertise within the OCE can enhance collaborative interactions and streamline administrative processes, facilitating rapid and thorough development and application review.

[14] PL 114-255. The 21st Century Cures Act. Title III Subtitle G Sec 3073: Establishment of Food and Drug Administration Intercenter Institutes.

Ultimately, this type of coordination will add efficiencies to the development of new technologies, bring a uniform approach to assessing benefits and risks, and allow cutting-edge treatments to reach patients as quickly as possible. But reaching this goal has been stymied by the current environment. The reality of lagging funding, the potential of a detrimental budget future, and the presence of a hiring freeze place this transformational opportunity at significant risk. As Congress resolves the budget for FY18, clarification that funds dedicated to the cancer moonshot can be transferred to the FDA for the OCE would provide important core support.

Despite challenges ahead that may weigh progress down, scientific advancement has brought us to a time of great opportunity. For the people who currently depend on safe and effective medicines, for those who are holding strong for the breakthroughs to come, and for every future patient, there isn't time to waste. The work that will be made possible through innovative policy like the 21st Century Cures Act will catalyze progress and improve lives and health of Americans. Building on these advancements, we urge Congress to swiftly pass this sixth reauthorization of PDUFA. In addition, to fully capitalize on this progress, and ensure that patients and physicians have access to the highest quality post-market evidence, new processes should be developed to maintain more up-to-date drug labels. Finally, for the programs of this proposed user fee agreement to succeed, the full budget for the FDA must be robust, and the capacity at which the agency can maintain and hire the best scientific minds must be unencumbered.

About Friends of Cancer Research

Friends of Cancer Research drives collaboration among partners from every healthcare sector to power advances in science, policy and regulation that speed life-saving treatments to patients. www.focr.org

Mr. Guthrie. Thank you. Thank you for your testimony, and I now recognize Ms. Holcombe for 5 minutes for your opening statement.

STATEMENT OF KAY HOLCOMBE

MS. HOLCOMBE. Mr. Vice Chairman, Ranking Member Green, and members of the subcommittee, Bio appreciates the opportunity to speak with you today about the sixth reauthorization of the Prescription Drug User Fee act. Let me begin by stating unequivocally that BIO strongly supports this PDUFA VI user fee agreement and its timely authorization.

Nearly 25 years ago, completing action begun by this committee, Congress passed the first PDUFA after agreeing with FDA and the biopharmaceutical industry that providing additional staff funded by user fees would help FDA review applications more quickly. You were shown to be spectacularly right. Today in this final year of PDUFA V, FDA is the most efficient drug regulatory agency in the world. American patients are the beneficiaries.

The success of PDUFA in bringing down the time of new drug review has led over the years to substantial expansion of the program in terms of the numbers and kinds of commitments FDA has made annually from increasing its efficiency in communicating with drug developers to enhancing its post-market surveillance and monitoring of drugs throughout their life cycles to applying best review practices across all review divisions to enhancing processes to review and approve therapies for rare diseases to executing systematic approaches to measuring the benefit-risk ratio of potential drugs and to seeking and incorporating patient perspectives in that assessment.

What has worked relative to review of applications has also made a difference in drug development. In PDUFA VI that is taken to a new level. FDA formal review time is the mere tip of the iceberg of time patients wait for new drugs. Review timelines are significant not only because they are short, but also because they are predictable and predictability is critical for companies making investment decisions. It would be highly desirable if the same sort of efficiency and predictability were achieved throughout drug development.

PDUFA VI builds on the proven premise that greater and more productive interaction between drug developers and FDA works. It leads to better outcomes and to more efficient development programs. A greater focus on drug development improvements in PDUFA VI is not at the sacrifice of what has been achieved for review times, 8 months for priority applications and 12 months for standard.

The PDUFA VI goals, including expanding expertise in diverse statistical methods, piloting innovative clinical trial designs and computer modeling and simulation, use of biomarkers as surrogate endpoints, and more frequent and appropriate use of real-world evidence or big data will transform drug development. All of these goals which attempt to bring 21st century science to the fore in this agreement will augment, not completely replace, tried and true methods of data collection. In the end, these new approaches will add to the old to make drug development more efficient while not compromising the statutory gold standard of substantial evidence of safety and effectiveness.

PDUFA VI also will take patient focused drug development to new levels. The message of these commitments is that the patient voice truly matters, in the beginning when early studies show a promising treatment and at the end when FDA is making its decision about a product's benefit and risk. PDUFA VI will bring the patient voice to the forefront, changing it from a voice with a compelling story to a voice that provides evidence, verifiable, valid evidence that is appropriate for the drug label.

Finally, Mr. Chairman, I want to emphasize how crucial it is that FDA has the ability to hire and retain the people it needs to carry out its PDUFA goals and to do that without jeopardizing the other significant parts of its public health mission. PDUFA is a carefully negotiated agreement that takes account of input from all stakeholders including FDA, industry, patient and consumer groups, and others. The key questions on the table are what needs to be changed or enhanced and what is the actual verifiable cost of achieving those goals?

The majority of costs paid by user fees are for personnel. This agreement is carefully crafted to ensure that FDA can bring those people on board who are needed to meet the goals, employees who costs are paid by user fees. In PDUFA VI, the annual hiring goals are included in the agreement. This allows the public a line of sight into whether goals may fall by the wayside as a result of an inability to hire.

Mr. Guthrie. Thank you. You need to summarize or is that your conclusion?

Ms. Holcombe. In conclusion, I want to reiterate BIO's strong support for this agreement. It satisfies our basic goals of financial transparency, long-term program viability, hiring and retention improvements to ensure stability and achieve the agreed-upon goals. The vision of PDUFA VI is the vision of 21st Century Cures. Put patient needs——

Mr. Guthrie. Thank you.

Ms. Holcombe [continuing]. For access to new medicines first.

[The prepared statement of Kay Holcombe follows:]

Testimony of Kay Holcombe, Senior Vice President, Science Policy, Biotechnology Innovation Organization

United States House of Representatives Energy and Commerce Committee, Subcommittee on Health Hearing on "Examining FDA's Prescription Drug User Fee Program"

March 22, 2017

Mr. Chairman, Ranking Member Green, and Members of the Subcommittee:

BIO appreciates the opportunity to speak with you today about the reauthorization of the Prescription Drug User Fee Act program (PDUFA). BIO strongly supports this fifth reauthorization of PDUFA and urges timely Congressional action.

I am Kay Holcombe, the Senior Vice President for Science Policy at BIO. BIO is the world's largest trade association representing biotechnology companies, academic institutions, state biotechnology centers, and related organizations across the United States and in more than

30 other nations. While our membership includes most of the large biopharmaceutical companies, the vast majority of our members are small biotechnology companies working on cutting-edge R&D. They have small staffs, no marketed products, and no profits, and they are heavily reliant on private capital to fund their work. They take enormous risks every day to develop the next generation of biomedical breakthroughs for the millions of patients suffering from diseases for which there are no effective cures or treatments today. BIO is proud of their innovative spirit and their dedication to alleviating human suffering.

All FDA stakeholders – the biopharmaceutical industry, patient and consumer advocates, health care providers, payers, and others in the healthcare system – recognize the importance of the PDUFA program. Many of them recall the time before enactment of PDFUA I in 1992, when FDA review times were lengthy and a high percentage of new drugs were on the market outside the United States before American patients had access to them. It was first at this Committee that FDA testified that review times could be reduced significantly if the agency could hire the additional staff, funded by user fees, needed to carry out the activities related to review of human drug applications more quickly.

PDUFA I proved this proposition. By the end of the five years of that first PDUFA program, review times had dropped by as much as three-fold. This significant improvement in review times has continued throughout the 24 years of PDUFA. Today, thanks to the resources PDUFA has provided FDA, U.S. patients are – in the vast majority of cases – the first in the world to have access to approved new drugs.

Formal FDA review time is, in fact, the shortest part of the process of moving a new therapy from its inception as a scientifically well-founded hypothesis to its use by patients. Today, it takes 10 to 12 to even 15 years and upwards of $2 billion to move a drug or biological product from a good idea to an approved product. During that lengthy period, unmet medical needs remain unmet and patients wait. Over the course of four previous PDUFA reauthorizations, the question has been raised as to whether and how the sorts of efficiencies that reduced review times also could reduce drug development times. How can FDA use PDUFA resources to address lengthy, expensive, risky drug development times?

PDUFA V, the program currently in place, was the first to include regulatory science initiatives – development of expertise in FDA to deal with cutting-edge technology and new ways of thinking about the studies and data associated with working toward approval of a new drug. PDUFA V provided funding for modest programs related to patient-focused drug development, the use of pharmacogenomics data, biomarkers as surrogate endpoints, patient-reported outcomes, and meta- analysis – some areas where additional expertise and resources could advance the science and the success rate. A key rationale for inclusion of those initiatives was that they are emerging areas in drug development that hold potential for reducing development times. Addressing drug development times would be a recurring theme entering this PDUFA reauthorization cycle.

Overall Goals for PDUFA VI

As BIO approached this reauthorization of PDUFA, we asked our member companies what they hoped to gain. We heard two themes: advance ways to reduce the time of drug development and ensure that PDUFA remains viable into the future. As to the former, our principal goals were to integrate the patient perspective in drug development; incorporate the use of innovative clinical trial designs, biomarkers as surrogate endpoints, and real-world evidence into acceptable approaches to drug development; and enhance some existing FDA processes, including the review of combination products that will be at the heart of personalized medicine. As to the viability of the PDUFA program, we sought to increase the transparency and accountability of PDUFA financial management and assure the long-term financial stability of the PDUFA program, including through a new time reporting system that would allow accurate capacity planning. Finally, but of primary importance, we sought to work with FDA to improve the agency's ability to attract, hire, and retain the numbers and kinds of employees it needs to do its job as efficiently and effectively as possible.

Program Sustainability and Financial Transparency

Since PDUFA finances and personnel form the foundation that keeps the PDUFA program viable, it is important to look at the situation as it exists today and what needs to be addressed. Since 2002, the PDUFA program has grown at an average of 11% per year; this is unsustainable moving into the future. Changes are needed that address the fee collection structure to increase efficiency and reduce administrative burdens for both FDA and companies. These include reducing the volatility of fee collections, eliminating complicated collection and other financial mechanisms that are difficult to administer, improving predictability, and reducing variation of collections year over year. Together, these changes will increase efficiency and reduce program growth rate substantially. Specifically, the PDUFA VI proposals would:

- limit the carryover balance levels, thus reducing possible over-collection of fees and the need for complicated administrative mechanisms to deal with such over-collections;
- eliminate supplement fees, which will further simplify fee collections;
- replace the current Product and Manufacturing fees with a new Program fee that will constitute 80% of the annual fee collections; and
- reduce the percentage that Application fees contribute to the total from the current 33% to 20%, thus mitigating the overall impact of this difficult-to-predict revenue source.

Increased financial transparency will provide a greater line of sight by Congress and the public into how PDUFA fees are collected and allocated and a more accurate picture of the costs associated with human drug review activities. This will be accomplished under PDUFA VI by improving resource management, thus allowing the public to know accurately how PDUFA fees are being used and to understand clearly the costs associated with human drug review related activities, and by providing a publicly available 5- year financial plan and annual updates of how the agency is executing against that plan. In both the development of the initial plan and throughout the remaining years of PDUFA VI, public input will be sought through public meetings and other mechanisms.

Transparency also will be increased as regards the calculation of the PDUFA workload. Until PDUFA VI, PDUFA fees have been adjusted annually by applying an inflation factor, which is straightforward and understandable, and a workload adjustor, which is neither. More than one outside consultant has stated that, while there is a clear need to apply an adjustment factor to account for differing workloads year over year, the particular adjustment factor was not a good one but was the only possibility unless there was systemic change in the way workload was measured. That systemic change is coming in PDUFA VI.

Beginning now, and through PDUFA VI, FDA will implement a new time reporting system, in which time and costs are measured on a continuous basis, rather than by sampling at pre-determined time periods throughout the year. This kind of system, used by multiple private sector organizations as well as in many government programs, provides significantly more accurate data than are now available on which to base workload calculations. FDA will be advised and assisted in establishing and executing the new system by an outside contractor with expertise in such systems. Progress toward this implementation and initiation of the new adjustment factor will be publicly available information, reported in the PDUFA annual Performance Report.

These more accurate time and cost data also will contribute to the ability to plan for future resource needs, contributing to the long-term sustainability of the PDUFA program. A capacity planning function will be established, which will allow FDA to assess in advance the number of staff that will be needed to assure a continuing efficient and effective human drug review program. Achievement of this goal is under way, with a third-party expert already working with the agency on determining the best approach to development and use of capacity planning.

Personnel Management

Hiring and retaining the expert staff essential to carrying out user-fee-funded activities is critical for PDUFA VI to work. Without the necessary number and kinds of staff, FDA simply cannot meet the performance goals for which user fees are intended. Problems with FDA recruitment and hiring have existed for years, for a number of reasons, including cumbersome hiring processes and pay scales that generally are lower than for similar positions in the private sector. The 21st Century Cures Act, from this Committee, addressed some of the issues that have hindered FDA's ability to attract, hire, and bring on board the kinds of senior scientific and medical staff needed. Those provisions will make a significant positive impact. In addition, under PDUFA VI FDA has committed to make changes in its internal personnel operations, including implementing a dedicated senior scientist recruiting function, increasing staff capacity to recruit and to process personnel actions in a timely way, and engaging the services of independent contractors to assist in these functions, advise the agency in best human resources practices, and evaluate and report annually and publicly on hiring and retention progress.

For the first time, hiring goals are included in detail in the PDUFA VI Performance Goals Letter, and achievement of these goals will be detailed in the annual PDUFA Performance Reports. Many of these changes already are under way. For example, FDA has begun the process of hiring staff to replenish the long-under-staffed Office of New Drugs, responsible for the review of all new drug and biologics applications. This hiring in FY 2017 is funded from PDUFA V amounts in the carryover balance. The balance exists as a result of earlier sequestration and continuing resolutions, which prevented the allocation of some PDUFA V resources before now. This hiring will continue in the first several years of PDUFA VI, along with hiring of additional staff essential to carry out the new performance goals agreed to between FDA and industry, in collaboration with other stakeholders such as patient, consumer, and provider organizations.

Over the course of PDUFA VI, the negotiated and agreed-upon number of FTEs (full-time equivalents) necessary to carry out the goals of PDUFA VI is 230, hired over years of the user fee agreement, FY 2018 to 2022. These include medical reviewers, pharmacologists, pharmacists, chemists and other scientific experts, biostatisticians, financial managers, and other essential staff. In each year's performance report, beginning in FY 2018, FDA will report on its progress in achieving the hiring goals specified in the PDUFA VI Goals Letter.

To summarize our views on the financial and hiring enhancements of PDUFA VI: BIO believes they are on target and essential to ensure both the long-term viability of this crucially important use fee program and to ensure that FDA is able to hire, bring on board, and retain the expert staff who are crucial for the agency to meet its PDUFA VI goals and, in general, to carry out its public health mission. We all have the same goals – ensuring that FDA-approved safe and effective therapies are available to patients as soon as possible. This Committee addressed them in 21st Century Cures; we add to that work through the PDUFA VI goals.

Making a Difference for Drug Development = Making a Difference for Patients

PDUFA VI promises to transform drug development. We believe FDA can and will deliver on this promise, provided they continue to have the ability to hire the additional people needed to carry out the historic commitments of this agreement.

In the beginning, the intention of prescription drug user fees was to improve the efficiency of FDA's review and reduce its time. That goal has been achieved. Today, the vast majority of new drugs are available to U.S. patients before they are available to patients anywhere else. FDA is the fastest and most efficient drug regulator in the world. All those who supported the establishment of the PDUFA program have been proven right. In August 1992, then-FDA Commissioner David Kessler made his first appeal to Congress in his testimony before this Committee, that if the agency had access to greater resources through a user fee program, review times could be reduced significantly. Industry, though with some skepticism, agreed. The Committee reported the first user fee bill shortly thereafter, with strong bipartisan support, and PDUFA was signed into law on October 19, 1992, by President George H.W. Bush. The rest is history.

Over the course of the four reauthorizations of PDUFA and as a result of user fees, we have seen review times drop dramatically from what they were before 1992, and we have seen other changes as well, such as enhancement in FDA's efficient and effective communication with applicants; augmentation of the agency's ability to monitor and assure the safety of products both pre- and post-market, throughout product life cycles, including establishment and use of the Sentinel program; adoption of best practices for scientific review and communication across all the review divisions in the Centers for Drugs and Biologics; establishment and implementation of regulatory science programs to deal more effectively with emerging areas of product research and development, such as the use of biomarkers, pharmacogenomic data, and patient-reported outcomes; and multiple other goals to ensure timely, efficient review. While all of these goals were being achieved, review timelines were not negatively affected. FDA consistently has met or exceeded its established goals of completing the review of Priority applications in eight months (many such priority applications are completed in fewer than eight months) and of Standard applications in 12 months. These timelines are now the global gold standard for regulatory efficiency. In the U.S. our economy has benefited from PDUFA, because drug and biologic applicants now have greater certainty of a reasonable timeline for completion of their applications. Most importantly, though, patients have benefited. Before PDUFA, U.S. patients legitimately could say that their counterparts elsewhere in the world had treatments available before they did. That largely is not the case anymore.

For nearly its entire history, PDUFA has been focused principally on the timeliness and efficiency of the formal FDA review process after an application has been submitted for approval. Yet FDA's application review time of less than 12 months pales by comparison to the 10 to 12 years on average that it takes to develop a drug – time before an application even is submitted to the FDA. Development of new medicines is a long and rigorous process, and it has become more costly and complex over the past decade – partly because the science is harder, and partly because the regulatory review process has not kept up with the advancing science.

The question facing PDUFA VI stakeholders and FDA was the question that faced this Committee as it embarked on 21st Century Cures: What can be done to change the course of drug development and to reduce the time it takes to get to that goal of submitting an application to FDA?

To tackle these questions, it was important to identify what new tools are available today that aid in drug development. Advances in biology have made miracles such as gene therapy more than a pipe dream or science fiction. Are there other advances that, if used to greater advantage, can accomplish the miraculous with respect to drug development?

The authors of 21st Century Cures and the PDUFA VI agreement independently recognized some of the same new tools and developed proposals and PDUFA VI commitments that would allow these tools to be used most effectively, with the goal of ensuring more timely availability of new drugs for patients by reducing the time and increasing the chance of success of drug development.

Key Drug Development Goals of PDUFA VI

Integrating the Patient Voice in Drug Development and Regulatory Decision-Making

One of the most important goals of PDUFA VI was building on the success of the PDUFA V Voice of the Patient program, in which public meetings brought FDA and patient representatives together so the agency and other stakeholders could hear how these patients perceived their condition, what they hoped for in terms of a "benefit" from a therapy, and how they viewed "risk." Those meetings, and the reports produced from them, were a positive step forward in terms of bringing these patient perceptions into the FDA determination of the benefit-risk calculus. Patients augmented that deliberation by adding the crucial patient perception dimension to an often largely mathematical and statistical evaluation. They also helped drug developers to understand better what patients viewed as their needs, so this could be taken into account when planning and executing a development program.

The next step in this approach is to engage patients and other stakeholders in another public process that will result in guidance, developed by FDA with stakeholder input, in a step-wise fashion. First, guidance will be developed regarding how to collect evidence-based and representative patient information. Next will be guidance on processes and approaches to determine what is most important to patients in terms of the impacts of their disease and potential impact of new treatments. This will be followed by guidance on how to measure impacts in a way that will facilitate meaningful patient input into the design of clinical trials. This is particularly important in light of the cost and length of clinical trials, the difficulty of enrolling sufficient numbers of patients, and the risk of patient drop-out, which can compromise or even negate the trial results. Finally, FDA will re-visit its existing guidance on patient-reported outcomes and address incorporating clinical outcome assessments into endpoints.

To accomplish these objectives, FDA will strengthen its staff capacity, including bringing on board experts in psychometrics and health outcomes research. These staff will be integrated into the review teams to ensure the engagement of patients and to consult with drug developers during their development programs.

Ultimately, the goal of good data collection, representative sampling, and appropriate use of data is to be able to include information on the drug label that can be used by prescribers, patients, and caregivers.

The drug label is the trusted source of information about the best and safest ways to use a drug. Reliable patient input into belongs in that label, and this PDUFA VI agreement will help make that happen.

Enhancing Benefit-Risk Assessment

FDA established a structured benefit-risk approach under PDUFA V. In PDUFA VI, implementation of this approach will be enhanced through one or more public meetings with and for stakeholders, and through development and publication of guidance on the use of the benefit-risk framework throughout the drug life cycle. The incorporation of patient perspectives will be a key part of these activities. An independent third party will evaluate the implementation of the benefit-risk framework and whether it is being implemented consistently across the review divisions. The importance of this goal is three-fold: first, it solidifies and evaluates the use of the benefit-risk framework, which allows greater transparency for all stakeholders into FDA's thinking about how to measure the potential benefits of a potential new drug against its known risks; second, it emphasizes the importance of patient input into this crucial decision; and, third, it helps drug developers use the benefit-risk assessment as a marker and a tool in the course of the development of a drug and throughout its lifecycle.

Enhancing Communication between FDA and Drug Sponsors

PDUFA VI builds on the enhanced communications program established under PDUFA V, which was intended to assure that sponsors were able to receive timely responses to inquiries that could be dealt with outside of the formal FDA-sponsor meeting process. Under PDUFA VI, a third party will evaluate how this program is proceeding, how such informal communications are handled across review divisions, and what best practices may be adopted across the board. A public meeting will allow stakeholders an opportunity for discussion and input into the evaluator's findings.

Using Drug Development Tools, including Biomarkers

In PDUFA VI, FDA is committed to enhancing biomarker qualification processes. In addition, the agency will implement a pilot program to seek and incorporate the input of external experts to assist in the qualification, to verify if the use of such outside experts can make the processes more timely and efficient. In addition, the agency will augment its staff capacity to conduct qualification of drug development tools, hold a public workshop particularly aimed at discussing nomenclature, standards, and elements of a biomarker qualification plan; publish guidance; and publish and update lists of qualified biomarkers and of pending applications. Significantly, FDA will establish a process for holding dedicated meetings with sponsors to discuss the use of biomarkers as surrogate endpoints. This will be a new meeting, additional to those meetings that all drug developers are entitled to have with FDA during their development programs.

Using Real-World Evidence

The Sentinel system, established by FDA in response to Congressional direction, is the source of enormous data regarding the health care and health outcomes of tens of millions of patients covered by several private insurance plans. FDA uses the system to search for safety signals that may lead to further investigations regarding the safety of marketed drug products. The system is supported by a number of sources, including user fees. Under PDUFA VI, prescription drug user fees will provide $50 million to continue to support the operation and use of Sentinel. FDA will work, during the course of PDUFA VI, to ensure that stakeholders, including industry, are well informed about how the agency is using the system and to seek additional ways to help others, beyond FDA, access this treasure trove of data while protecting any patient and drug sponsor confidential information.

In addition to the data available through Sentinel, there are multiple other sources of "real-world evidence" that currently are seen primarily as a potential source of drug safety information. Under PDUFA VI, FDA will hold a public meeting and, based on that input, develop pilot studies or related activities to determine other uses of such real-world data in regulatory decision-making. One possibility is that large data bases could be used as a source of information that could augment other sponsor-developed data in applications for approval of a new indication for an already approved drug. Another possible use is for the fulfillment of post-marketing requirements associated with newly marketed drugs.

Data are everywhere. The question PDUFA VI will begin to answer is how such data can be harnessed and used effectively to advance, enhance, and reduce the time of drug development.

Improving the Review of Combination Products

Combination products – which join two drugs, a drug and a biologic, or a drug or biologic and a medical device, commonly a diagnostic test – pose some unique challenges to developers. Streamlining and better assignment of roles and responsibilities at FDA could help address these challenges and advance these products, which many see as a wave of the future. For example, personalized medicine is highly dependent on identifying, often through a diagnostic test, patients who will benefit from a particular drug and those who are likely not to benefit, or who may be subject to greater risk. Such advancements will not only benefit patients, but also facilitate the broader move toward a more cost-effective healthcare system.

The challenges that have been identified as slowing the review of such products include the decision as to which FDA Center has primary or lead responsibility, which Center has decision-making authority, and how to speed the work of the "other" Center that may not have a user fee goal impetus to make a particular application a priority. PDUFA VI will address these challenges in several ways. First, staff capacity and training will be increased in all three medical product Centers, the Centers for Drugs, Biologics, and Devices. PDUFA funds will be used for bringing staff on board in all three Centers. Second, performance goals will be established specific to combination products and will be phased in over the course of the 5 years of PDUFA VI. Submission procedures and guidance related to unique features of combination products will be developed and published.

Using Innovative Clinical Trial Designs

Clinical trials are the most costly and difficult parts of drug development, and their design, enrollment, and execution can add extraordinarily to the time of drug development. Many experts in trial design have argued that the "traditional" randomized, double-blind, controlled trial is not always the most efficient or necessary approach. With new ways of thinking, and given new approaches to statistical analysis, are there better ways to do trials without losing their validity, their amenability to appropriate data analysis, and, thus, their contribution to the most appropriate regulatory decision?

In PDUFA VI, FDA is committed to beginning to answer that question. First, additional FDA staff, particularly additional biostatisticians, and especially those with training and expertise in "non-traditional" statistical analysis, will be added. FDA will hold a public workshop on innovative trial design and will publish guidance on adaptive trials. Finally, and of particular significance for moving this idea forward, FDA will conduct a pilot program focused on innovative trial designs. This program will be voluntary – i.e., companies may opt in to the program and, in exchange for their participation, will be given two meetings with FDA to discuss the proposed trial design and its execution, to enhance the likelihood of success of the development program. Companies in the program will agree to allow FDA to discuss the trial design as a case study at a subsequent public workshop or in guidance (protecting all company-specific confidential information). Participation in the pilot program is voluntary, but the hope is that there will be strong participation, so the ability for others to learn from case studies will "raise all boats," expand the use of innovative trials, and contribute to reducing the time and cost of clinical trials.

Using Model-Informed Drug Development (MIDD)

Biological and statistical modeling can contribute greatly to a knowledge base that can advance drug development, reduce the time of development, and allow development to proceed even in cases where clinical data may be limited. FDA will explore the use of MIDD through both increasing its staff capabilities and establishing a voluntary pilot program similar to that for innovative clinical trial design. In addition, the agency will hold workshops to identify best practices for various types of modeling and publish guidance based on its findings through the workshops and in the pilot program. Modeling informs development, and is not intended as a complete substitute for clinical data. Part of the importance of this program is that it can determine how modeling can assist in moving forward a significant development program where clinical data are limited. Modeling or simulation would not be the only source of data in any program of developing a human drug.

Continuing and Enhancing Successful Programs

PDUFA VI will continue and enhance its efforts related to the highly successful Breakthrough Therapy program, which has shown the power of enhanced communication between FDA and sponsors to speed drug development for exciting new products; augment its capacity and enhance its processes for reviewing applications for rare disease therapies, to continue its record of success in prioritizing these applications based on the high unmet medical need of patients with rare diseases; and continue and build on the successful New Molecular Entity (NME) review program, which has accomplished its goal of increasing the number of products approved after only one cycle of review. All of these programs are resulting in reducing the time of drug development. All of them are verified and verifiable successes.

PDUFA VI and 21st Century Cures: Great Minds Think Alike

When this Committee embarked in a bipartisan effort to learn how to advance science and regulation in ways that would lead to better, healthier lives for patients, it identified – through consultation with experts around the country, including patients, caregivers, regulators and former regulators, industry, and many others – it achieved the near-impossible. It found suggestions common to many disparate stakeholders for improving the processes of basic research that are fundamental to understanding disease and treating it and for improving the processes of translating that research into real products that are safe and effective and can be made available to patients. In the latter category were suggestions that focused on improving drug development timelines through applying new tools and new ideas and encouraging and directing FDA to incorporate those into its thinking when reviewing applications.

Perhaps not surprisingly, some of these tools and ideas also came into the discussions between FDA and stakeholders in developing the PDUFA VI agreement. The skeptical might worry that such an overlap of ideas in two separate and very different contexts is a recipe for disaster. Not so. In fact, there is the best sort of overlap between the provisions of 21st Century Cures and PDUFA VI – the kind that results in each enhancing the other. A few examples, not an exhaustive list, are illustrative.

Biomarkers

A word that has, over the last two years, come into the lexicon of people who never thought of a biomarker before – are a focus both of PDUFA VI and of 21st Century Cures. The Act and PDUFA VI are complementary, in terms of ensuring that FDA has and uses effectively an efficient process for qualifying biomarkers; publishes guidance to help applicants for biomarker qualification understand the taxonomy and data standards; makes public a list of qualified biomarkers and pending applications; and engages external experts in biomarker qualification.

Patient-Focused Drug Development

In this area as well, it is clear that there is near-universal agreement on the need to do more, and in a more systematic way, to incorporate the patient perspective into drug development and regulatory decision-making. Guidance development, public meetings, development of methods and standards for collecting information and data, and use of patient perception and experience information in the FDA regulatory decision about the benefits and risks of a drug are all elements of both 21st Century Cures and the PDUFA VI agreement.

Real-World Evidence

There is considerable overlap between the provisions of 21st Century Cures and PDUFA VI. 21st Century Cures provides helpful context for the work under PDUFA VI, and provisions of the two that differ are easily harmonized.

Innovative Trial Design

While 21st Century Cures focuses on adaptive trials and Bayesian approaches, PDUFA VI takes a broader approach, opening its pilot program to other trial designs while also highlighting adaptive trials and Bayesian approaches. Public processes, including workshops, and guidance development are parts of both.

In short, it surely is the case, looking at PDUFA VI and 21st Century Cures together, that there is broad agreement about what is needed to reduce the time of drug development.

BIO strongly supported and applauds the enactment of 21st Century Cures, as we strongly support the PDUFA VI negotiated agreement. We believe that, together, these two efforts will make a difference for patients.

BIO urges Congress to act swiftly to move the PDUFA VI reauthorization forward. This agreement, negotiated between FDA and the biopharmaceutical industry with input and support from multiple other stakeholders, positively advances our shared goal of making safe and effective treatments available to patients as efficiently and quickly as possible.

Thank you for the opportunity to present our views today. I am happy to answer any questions you may have.

Mr. Guthrie. Thank you very much. Now Dr. Pritchett, you are recognized for 5 minutes for opening statement.

STATEMENT OF ANNE PRITCHETT

Ms. Pritchett. Good morning, Vice Chairman Guthrie, Ranking Member Green, and members of the subcommittee. I am please to appear before you to provide PhRMA's perspective on the timely reauthorization of PDUFA. PhRMA, as you know, represents the country's leading innovative biopharmaceutical research companies which are devoted to developing new medicines that enable patients to live longer, healthier, and more productive lives. We appreciate the opportunity to testify and share our views on PDUFA VI.

For over 2 decades, PDUFA has helped to bring innovative medicines to patients by providing greater clarity and predictability in the science-based drug review process. Today, I just want to briefly share PhRMA's perspective on the PDUFA program and key elements of the PDUFA VI agreement.

First, I just want to note that we view user fees as an important mechanism to support the critical work of the FDA and human drug review process, and note as a result of this program over 1,500 new drugs and biologics have been approved since 1992. The number of new medicines being approved on their first review cycle is at a historic high, and as we heard earlier, the review times have dramatically dropped by more than half since the 1990s as a result of this agreement.

As a result of PDUFA, the U.S. leads the world in the introduction of new medicines and is a global leader in biopharmaceutical R&D. I would note at a time when other countries are seeking to attract and grow their own biopharmaceutical presence due to its far-reaching economic impacts, it is more critical than ever that we ensure that the U.S. retains its competitive advantages which includes a science-based gold standard regulatory system in the FDA, one that facilitates the ability of our industry to harness the latest scientific and technological advances and to translate those into new treatments and cures for patients.

I would note that PDUFA VI is a result of extensive negotiations between the FDA and the innovative biopharmaceutical industry and it really includes unprecedented input across all stakeholders. Patients and patient advocates in particular played an important role by providing input on potential PDUFA VI goals through for- mal stakeholder meetings with the agency as well as frequent interactions with industry, and that feedback is reflected in several of the provisions. I would note failure to reauthorize

PDUFA in a timely manner would obviously negatively impact the FDA's ability to carry out its important role in fostering the introduction of new medicines to patients.

And I want to briefly touch on some key elements of the agreement. First, obviously PDUFA VI facilitates science-based integration of the patient perspective into the development and regulatory review of innovative medicines. Over the course of PDUFA VI, FDA will be holding a number of workshops to gather stakeholder input to inform a range of guidances that are focused on how do we better incorporate the patient element into all stages of drug development and review.

Second, PDUFA VI enhances the FDA's access to the tools, processes, and expertise necessary to ensure that the FDA is ready for the 21st century, the latest scientific advances in drug development and regulation. Specifically, as mentioned by other witnesses, there will be an increase in the FDA's capacity to qualify biomarkers. The agreement advances the use of real-world evidence building on 21st Century Cures facilitates the appropriate use of innovative clinical trial approaches.

Third, PDUFA VI will accelerate the development and availability of new medicines to patients while providing the scientific and regulatory predictability that will foster a continued biopharmaceutical innovation. PDUFA VI not only builds upon the highly successful new molecular entity review program, which has led to shorter review times and an increase in first cycle reviews, but it builds upon it by incorporating additional metrics.

Fourth, PDUFA ensures that the FDA will be able to hire and maintain a strong scientific medical and regulatory workforce to advance its public health mission. For the first time, PDUFA VI includes detailed hiring goals and includes dedicated resources for the recruitment and retention of a world-class scientific workforce. And I would note it also includes independent outside consultants to help facilitate the agency in developing a comprehensive hiring strategy.

And finally, the agreement builds on key provisions of the 21st Century Cures Act by further advancing real-world evidence, incorporating that into a structured benefit-risk framework, patient-focused drug development, biomarker qualification, as well as includes a number of improvements to combination product review.

I want to conclude by saying PhRMA and its member companies we are committed to working closely with the FDA, your committee, Congress, and all stakeholders to ensure the continued success of PDUFA in bringing safe and effective innovative medicines forward to address unmet medical needs for all patients. We believe that moving all of the UFA's forward in a timely manner is important to supporting the FDA's mission of protecting public health and promoting innovation, as well as critical to supporting our shared goals of fostering continued competition and innovation. Thank you for the opportunity to testify today.

[The prepared statement of Anne Pritchett follows:]

Testimony of Anne Pritchett, PhD, Vice President, Policy and Research, Pharmaceutical Research and Manufacturers of America (PhRMA)

Before the U.S. House of Representatives, Energy and Commerce Committee Subcommittee on Health Hearing on "Examining FDA's Prescription Drug User Fee Program"

March 22, 2017

Good afternoon Chairman Burgess, Ranking Member Green, and the Members of the Subcommittee:

My name is Anne Pritchett, Vice President, Policy and Research, at the Pharmaceutical Research and Manufacturers of America (PhRMA). PhRMA represents the country's leading innovative biopharmaceutical research companies, which are devoted to developing medicines that enable patients to live longer, healthier and more productive lives. Since 2000, PhRMA member companies have invested more than half a trillion dollars in the search for new treatments and cures, including $59.6 billion in 2015 alone.

I am pleased to appear before you to provide PhRMA's perspective on the importance of the Prescription Drug User Fee Act (PDUFA) and its timely reauthorization. As you know PhRMA served as industry's principal negotiators with FDA for the PDUFA VI agreement. Our members are committed to the research and development of new therapies that enable patients today to live longer, healthier and more productive lives and through a robust pipeline of more than 7,000 investigational medicines, providing patients with hope for the treatments and cures of tomorrow.

Today, I will briefly speak to PhRMA's perspective on the successes of the PDUFA program and key elements of the PDUFA VI agreement.

Perspectives on the Success of the PDUFA Program

In the midst of the HIV/AIDS crisis of the 1980s, the United States lagged behind other countries in the review and approval of new medicines. The FDA faced a significant backlog in the regulatory review of new drug applications and was unable to keep pace with the workload related to the human drug review program. An average FDA review time of approximately 29 months[15] meant that in many instances new medicines were approved in other countries, months or years before they were available in the United States. This unacceptable delay compelled the patient advocacy community to catalyze a nationwide demand for faster review of drug applications. As a result, the first PDUFA was passed in 1992, giving the FDA the additional resources needed – through the collection of user fees – to improve application review times.

For nearly twenty-five years, PDUFA has provided much needed resources to the FDA's human drug review program that has resulted in greater certainty and predictability for patients who depend on safe and effective innovative medicines. PDUFA VI builds upon the successes of previous PDUFA agreements with continued focus on ensuring patient safety, maintaining the FDA's high standards for regulatory review, and, ultimately, promoting timely access to safe and effective innovative

[15] U.S. Food and Drug Administration (FDA), FY1995 Performance Report to the President and Congress for the Prescription Drug User Fee Act. www.fda.gov/AboutFDA/ReportsManualsForms/Reports/UserFeeReports/PerformanceReports/ucm117257.htm.

medicines, including treatments for patients with rare, serious, or life-threatening diseases.

The PDUFA program has produced positive and tangible results that matter to patients, ensuring that FDA's review process for new medicines keeps pace with biopharmaceutical innovation:

- FDA has approved over 1,500 new drugs and biologics since 1992, including treatments for cancer, cardiovascular, neurological, infectious and rare diseases.[16]
- The number of new medicines being approved on their first review cycle is at a historic high, including approvals for new medicines to treat rare diseases.[17]
- Review times for drug applications have dropped by nearly 55%. The median approval time for standard applications has decreased from 22.1 months in 1993 to an estimated 10 months in 2015.[18] The median approval time for priority applications has similarly decreased from 13.2 months in 1993 to an estimated 7.9 months in 2014.[19]

As a result of PDUFA, the "drug lag" between the United States and the rest of the world has been eliminated, and the United States leads the world in the introduction of new medicines without compromising FDA's appropriately high safety or efficacy standards. At a time when the economic competitiveness of our nation is recognized to be strongly rooted in our capacity to advance innovation-based industries, PDUFA VI is

[16] U.S. Food and Drug Administration (FDA), PDUFA Background and Reauthorization Process (Presentation by Theresa Mullin). 15 July 2015 http://www.fda.gov/downloads/ForIndustry/UserFees/PrescriptionDrugUserFee/UCM455134.pdf

[17] John Jenkins, FDA. CDER New Drug Review: 2015 Update (Presentation). 14 December 2015 http://www.fda.gov/downloads/AboutFDA/CentersOffices/OfficeofMedicalProductsandTobacco/CDER/UCM477020.pdf

[18] FDA, FY2015 Performance Report to the President and Congress for the Prescription Drug User Fee Act, http://www.fda.gov/downloads/AboutFDA/ReportsManualsForms/ Reports/UserFeeReports/PerformanceReports/UCM497750.pdf

[19] FDA, FY2015 Performance Report to the President and Congress for the Prescription Drug User Fee Act, http://www.fda.gov/downloads/AboutFDA/ ReportsManualsForms/ Reports/UserFeeReports/PerformanceReports/UCM497750.pdf

critical to providing the capabilities and efficiencies needed to encourage the significant R&D investments made by biopharmaceutical companies in the U.S.

Key Elements of PDUFA VI

The PDUFA VI agreement will help ensure the long-term stability of the user fee program, provide necessary resources and enhancements to FDA's human drug review program, and strengthen the scientific capabilities of the agency. Specifically, PDUFA VI will:

- Create efficiencies that can accelerate the development and availability of new medicines to patients, while providing greater predictability that will continue to foster biopharmaceutical innovation.
- Enhance the FDA's access to the tools, processes, and expertise necessary to keep pace with the latest scientific advances in drug development and regulation.
- Facilitate the systematic integration of the patient perspective into the development and regulatory review of innovative medicines.
- Ensure that FDA can hire and retain a strong scientific and medical workforce to advance its public health mission.

The PDUFA VI agreement strengthens pre-market review and post-market safety, enhances FDA's regulatory decision tools, and promotes financial accountability and capacity planning. We have identified some of the important provisions outlined in the agreement that will help to speed drug development, streamline the review process, and provide more options to innovative medicines for patients.

Improvements to Pre-Market Review and Post-Market Safety

As a focal point of PDUFA V, the New Molecular Entity (NME) Review Program has been very successful, as review times have been reduced, first cycle approvals have increased and the predictability for sponsors and patients has been strengthened through enhanced communication during the review period. PDUFA VI not only continues the NME Review Program, but will also build upon it by incorporating additional metrics to enhance the drug review and approval process. As part of the review, FDA will provide a timeline for drug scheduling recommendations during the pre-submission meeting and updates on these activities during the Mid- and Late-cycle Review meetings. In addition, FDA will update the Good Review Management Principles and Practices (GRMPs) guidance to include review activities not currently associated with specific PDUFA goals.

Under the PDUFA program, FDA and industry have worked together to ensure that meetings during the drug development phase are as efficient, substantive, and timely as possible. PDUFA VI will provide additional time for FDA's review of meeting materials for Type B and Type C meetings, while also providing sponsors with responses to their questions 5 days in advance for scheduled meetings. These changes will lead to more substantive engagements between FDA and sponsors and reduce the need for multiple meetings. This will allow for drug development programs to proceed in a timelier manner and expedite availability to new medicines for patients.

As a cornerstone of the PDUFA V agreement, the breakthrough therapy program has been a profound success. The response to the program has been remarkable—a sign of the swift pace of new scientific advances—and substantially more resource intensive for FDA to manage than anticipated. No additional resources were provided for this function in PDUFA V. PDUFA VI will dedicate significant new resources to the program to ensure that the workload is manageable and patients continue to gain expedited access to treatments for serious and life-threatening diseases that are currently without adequate treatment options.

The PDUFA program dedicates substantial resources to help ensure the safety of medicines when they are on the market. PDUFA VI will expand these efforts by providing significant resources to enhance the FDA's ability to review, track, and communicate important post- market safety information to patients, physicians, industry, and key stakeholders.

Enhancing FDA's Regulatory Decision-Making Tools

Patients and patient advocates played an important role in the PDUFA VI reauthorization process by providing input on potential PDUFA VI goals through formal stakeholder meetings with the agency and frequent interactions with industry. Patient group feedback is reflected throughout the PDUFA VI agreement. In particular, two provisions bring the patient voice directly into the development and review process:

- PDUFA VI will strengthen the FDA's capacity and capability to advance the science of patient input in the drug development and regulatory review process, including the use of patient-reported outcomes measures.
- Over the course of PDUFA VI, FDA will conduct a series of public workshops to gather stakeholder input to inform several guidances related to patient-focused drug development, the use of patient-reported outcomes, and the structured assessment of the benefits and risks of new medicines. Facilitating the development and application of scientific methods that incorporate the patient perspective into drug development will help ensure that medicines better reflect measures that are meaningful to patients.

PDUFA VI will also help facilitate the appropriate use of innovative clinical trials designs, including convening a workshop, publishing draft guidance, and conducting a voluntary pilot program. Innovative clinical trial approaches have the potential to enhance the efficiency of the drug development and regulatory review process, and help accelerate patient access to safe and effective new medicines.

"Model-informed drug development" and related statistical and modeling approaches have the potential to accelerate the development and availability of innovative medicines. PDUFA VI will establish processes to allow for the use of model-informed drug development to help reduce drug development and review times to make the interpretation of data more efficient while protecting patient safety.

PDUFA VI will increase staff capacity and resources for the qualification of biomarkers, including piloting approaches to engaging external experts in FDA's qualification process. As biomarker science has been progressing faster than regulatory acceptance, it is important that we shorten the time between biomarker discovery and assimilation into practice. A number of aspects of PDUFA VI seek to address this:

- FDA will hold a public workshop on biomarker qualification and publish guidance documents to provide all stakeholders, including academia, patient groups and biopharmaceutical companies, with further clarity on the data necessary to qualify a biomarker.
- A dedicated process will be created for scientific consultation between the Agency and sponsors for drug development programs that plan to use a biomarker as a novel surrogate endpoint.

Real-world evidence provides a valuable source of information about the safety and effectiveness of a medicine in a broader population beyond that studied in clinical trials. Advancing the science of using real-world evidence in regulatory decision-making, including studies based on electronic medical records and patient registries may accelerate the clinical development of additional uses for a medicine as well as the assessment of the benefits and risks of medicines. PDUFA VI will advance the potential use of real-world evidence for regulatory decision-making through public workshops with key stakeholders, pilot studies with sponsors, and the publication of guidance on how real-world evidence can contribute to the assessment of the safety and effectiveness of medicines.

Promoting Financial Accountability and Capacity Planning

The PDUFA VI agreement supports common sense financial reforms that provide greater predictability for the Agency. These reforms include reducing FDA's administrative burden and operating expenses for the PDUFA program without compromising the human drug review program performance, regulatory review standards, or patient safety. PDUFA VI reallocates the fee collection structure of the program, eliminating the establishment fee and providing more revenue through approved products, which enhances predictability, improves strategic planning, and provides better management of Agency resources.

PDUFA VI modernizes FDA's human resource capacity and capabilities to provide more accountability to stakeholders, including patients. FDA will implement a full time reporting system and establish a professional capacity planning function to better track workload, identify areas of need, and help reallocate resources when necessary. PDUFA VI will also provide resources for an independent contractor to assess the program and help to implement best practices to ensure the program remains adequately and appropriately funded for the future. Determining the most appropriate fee levels and ensuring the resources are most efficiently being utilized will provide FDA with the tools to further improve their capabilities as well as continue to ensure access for new products.

In order for FDA to have the ability to perform its duties of delivering safe and effective new medicines to patients and ensure the continued regulation of products throughout their lifecycle, it is imperative the Agency has the appropriate staff and expertise available to them. The human drug review program at FDA has been understaffed and has lacked certain scientific capabilities needed to fully achieve its goals. PDUFA VI will address this issue through providing dedicated resources for recruiting and retaining a world-class scientific and medical workforce, providing independent outside consultants to work with the Agency on a comprehensive hiring strategy, and for the first time including hiring goals within the agreement. These provisions will help ensure FDA is delivering new medicines to patients in a timely manner, and that they are prepared for the increasingly complex drug development and review challenges of the 21st Century.

Conclusion

At a time when the U.S medical innovation ecosystem is facing severe strains and increased global competition, it is imperative that the FDA is equipped to help us deliver the next generation of new treatments and cures to meet patients' unmet medical needs. PDUFA VI will help the FDA ensure that patients receive effective and lifesaving drugs, while maintaining the United States' global leadership in biomedical innovation.

PhRMA and its member companies are committed to working closely with FDA, and all stakeholders, to insure the continued success of PDUFA in bringing safe, effective innovative medicines forward to address unmet medical needs for all patients. PhRMA therefore urges Congress to reauthorize PDUFA in a timely manner to ensure the new enhancements are implemented as quickly as possible and protect against any disruptions to this important program.

PhRMA applauds your continued commitment to ensuring the long-term sustainability of the FDA's human drug review program and to continuing to strengthen the agency's capabilities in areas critical to keeping pace with the latest scientific advances in drug development and regulation. We look forward to continuing to work with the Subcommittee, members of Congress, and other stakeholders on these important issues. Thank you for the opportunity to provide this testimony.

Mr. Guthrie. Thank you all for your testimony, and we will now move into the question and answer portion for our second panel. And I will begin the questioning and recognize myself for 5 minutes.

First, I would like to request unanimous consent for entering the following statements in the record: the Rare Disease Legislative Advocates, the RDLA blog, PDUFA RDLA, Congress Begins Process of Reauthorizing Prescription Drug User Fee Act; a letter from the Epilepsy Foundation, letter; number three, National Venture Capital Association blog post on PDUFA; and four pieces I am asking to enter into the record, National Organization for Rare Diseases and Friends of Cancer Research joint statement on PDUFA.

Mr. Green. No objection.

Mr. Guthrie. No objection, so ordered.

[The information appears at the conclusion of the hearing.]

Mr. Guthrie. So Mr. Allen, actually Mr. Sarbanes was talking about this earlier with Dr. Woodcock, and where I kind of wanted to look at about labeling. And after a drug is approved, more and more information is often learned about it. This can include new uses, more tolerable doses, et cetera. And for cancer drugs, can you talk about the disparity between the information in products labeling and how the drug is actually being prescribed and administered by oncologists?

Mr. Allen. Sure. So typically a manufacturer would, if they are pursuing an additional indication for a drug, would take it and submit it through the supplemental new drug application at the FDA for that information to be evaluated. But in some instances like I mentioned, when a drug is off patent or perhaps even for a particularly rare population where a clinical trial is difficult or infeasible, or in some cases because the drug has been on the market for so long may be unethical, the label oftentimes doesn't reflect the practice and the use of that drug over time.

And what we found by comparing the FDA labels to practice guidelines that are constructed by medical oncologists is that the uses that are recommended by expert oncologists are usually far beyond that of what is contained in the FDA label. So the question is, should the product label have a role in the agency which we trust to evaluate medicines for them to get on the market, should they have a more active role in looking at potential label modifications further down the life cycle of the drug to ensure it is supported by the highest quality evidence.

Mr. Guthrie. Do you think FDA needs to clarify when and how companies can provide such information?

Mr. Allen. In terms of when it can be supplied to them? Mr. GUTHRIE. Yes.

Mr. Allen. I think it could——

Mr. Guthrie. When it needs to be.

Mr. Allen. The agency certainly does in terms of safety, but the same mechanisms aren't in place with regards to alternative uses. So one could imagine that perhaps it is worth having a longer discussion about the ability for over a certain period of time perhaps after the patent expires that there be some process for review of post-market evidence in order to make sure that the way the drug is being used is supported by the highest quality of evidence, so the people who are prescribing and using it are able to tell the difference between what is high quality and what is just an anecdotal use.

Mr. Guthrie. OK. And I had another question, but I think you did answer it that do you believe FDA should play a more active role in updating product labeling, and you answered that actually when you answered the first question.

Mr. Allen. Yes. I think it is worth a longer conversation because obviously there are resource implications. But given the oncology anyway there are highly qualified professional guidelines that might help the FDA conduct post-market analyses when it is appropriate to review a growing body of evidence.

Mr. Guthrie. Right. Yes, that is something that we just need to work to make sure we can clarify that because I think Dr. Woodcock was sharing similar to that when she was talking to Mr. Sarbanes about, some oncologists has a different tumor that this actually has effect for and works for and would be logical to use, but we need to make sure that it can be done through the process.

So thanks for your testimony, and actually I will yield back my extra minute and I will yield to Mr. Green, 5 minutes for questions.

Mr. Green. Thank you, Mr. Chairman.

Ms. Holcombe, current statute outlines a detailed process for reauthorization of the PDUFA. The FDA is charged not only with negotiating with the industry to develop recommendations, but also to solicit public input and hold public hearings and consult periodically with Congress and patients and consumer groups, among others. The recommendations that are a result of this process must also be available publicly for the public comment and ultimately required by statute to be transmitted to Congress by January 15th of this year. The process that led to the ultimate transmission of FDA PDUFA VI recommendations kicked off nearly 2 years ago in July of '15.

Ms. Holcombe, can you further discuss industry's role in the reauthorization of PDUFA and particularly the timeline for these activities?

Ms. Holcombe. So as you point out, Mr. Green, this process began in July of 2015 with a public meeting at which all stakeholders were provided an opportunity to testify, and industry took advantage of that opportunity and presented our views about the importance of PDUFA in general and about some specific enhancements to the program that we would be seeking in our negotiations with FDA. Those negotiations kicked off approximately 2 months later and lasted then for over 12 additional months and were intensively focused on the calculation of what could be done and how much it would cost to do each one of those things.

And both FDA and industry put ideas on the table, and those ideas were frequently, if not every single time, informed by the input of other meetings that were going on simultaneously with patients in the other groups that you mentioned, so it was a very long process and I would say mathematically and statistically a very precise process.

Mr. Green. Well, since this is our sixth time on it, hopefully we learn something every time.

Ms. Holcombe. Well, we are getting faster.

Mr. Green. OK. The statute requires that a recommendation be transmitted to Congress no later than July 15th of '17, a deadline they met. Does the statute allow the FDA to transmit recommendations for reauthorization at an alternative date?

Ms. Holcombe. Not that I am aware of.

Mr. Green. OK. PDUFA expires on September 30th of '17. What would be the impact for your member companies if Congress did not pass the reauthorization of PDUFA before the September 30th deadline?

Ms. Holcombe. I think we would describe the implications as titanic in nature. FDA would be required, if this were not reauthorized, to reduce its force by probably in the Drug Center alone about 5,000-plus individuals, and those are the people who review our applications. But even more importantly than the review of applications, which as we have all said today is merely the tip of the iceberg of our process of drug development, it would absolutely disable any process that FDA has for talking to us during drug development about how to be more successful in our program.

Mr. Green. Do you support and your industry support PDUFA VI recommendations as transmitted to Congress?

Ms. Holcombe. Yes, we do.

Mr. Green. OK. You note in your testimony that the drug development process, the most time-intensive part of bringing a drug to market, it is my understanding that on average it takes between 10 to 12 years to develop a drug. Recognizing this, we included in the 21st Century Cures a revision that would have FDA host a public workshop and issue guidance on innovative trials and designs and approaches.

Would you please explain further how innovative trial designs may help your member companies in bringing treatments to market quicker and, in addition, would you discuss how PDUFA VI builds off of the Cures' effort to support the use of innovative drug trial designs?

Ms. Holcombe. Yes. So as my testimony pointed out great minds think alike, and we in the industry as well as FDA itself agreed a hundred percent with you in your identification in 21st Century Cures of the importance of thinking of different ways to do clinical trials than the traditional way of randomized controlled trials.

Often clinical trials have to enroll many, many people and they take a long time. And as Dr. Woodcock pointed out, they often have high dropout rates. Patients can't stay in them, and these cause drugs to fail and at great expense to companies that are developing them. So innovative ways of thinking, creative ways of thinking could we do trials differently and therefore make them shorter and smaller but still come out with the substantial evidence of safety and effectiveness that we all need to have and the answer to that is yes, we can.

Mr. Green. OK. Mr. Chairman, I know my time has expired. And Mr. Allen, I would like to submit some more questions to you, but obviously

FDA is working with you on the off-label usage that practitioners learn, and we need to be able to learn what they are learning so we can actually make those pharmaceuticals available and go back through the FDA process as brief as we could do to make sure those cures are there. So thank you, Mr. Chairman.

Mr. Guthrie. Thank you. Thank you. The gentleman's time has expired. Dr. Bucshon, you are recognized for 5 minutes for questions.

Mr. Bucshon. Thank you, Mr. Chairman. First of all, I mean, I also want to go on the record saying I have concerns about the budget proposal as it relates to research, the NIH and above. I don't think that is a partisan issue.

The question I have is as we transition to new models to approve medicines we have been talking about that whether that is changes in clinical trials or other things, how do you see the legal environment evolving to allow this to happen? I will start with Dr. Pritchett. Because, I mean all of us are realists. I was a medical doctor before, as you transition to a new way to approve a product there is going to be people out there that are looking to throw a wrench into the gears by saying it didn't prove what it was supposed to prove and that is why my particular client has been hurt. And so I mean there are legal ramifications of trying to do this also, any thoughts?

Ms. Pritchett. So I think as I understand your question, as we think about looking at innovative, new approaches to clinical trials, collection of real-world evidence and how do we apply this to drug development and then how do we ensure that we are using them in a robust way so that we are reducing any potential concerns related to liability, ensuring that we aren't approving medications without appropriate evidence——

Mr. Bucshon. Essentially that is the question, because that is one of the things that drives up costs of drug approvals. Everybody has to look at those issues, but a percentage of the drug costs are because of these type of issues. My question would be basically is, I mean, yes, what are our thoughts about that? Do we need, I mean obviously we are working on tort reform in other areas. Any thoughts on that process as it relates to the drug product development?

Ms. Pritchett. So I am not prepared to discuss that today. We would be happy to come back and have further discussions with you. I would note that as we look at the PDUFA process, part of the engagement by FDA in providing very clear guidances to industry is to help avert any potential concerns from a liability perspective, et cetera, but I think this is an important topic that we would welcome to have further discussion.

Mr. Bucshon. OK, because I could see that the FDA and others very quickly retract their thoughts on these things as soon as we have some big class action lawsuit against the FDA and everybody else.

Ms. Pritchett. I think that is a very important issue that you are raising and we would greatly appreciate coming back and having further discussion on that topic. I appreciate you raising it.

Mr. Bucshon. OK, great, any other comments from the other panelists?

Ms. Holcombe. I think one of the important things to recognize about PDUFA VI is that in some respects takes account of this type of concern by initiating under PDUFA VI pilot programs, where the agency and the industry are going to work together to pilot these various trial designs or model-informed drug development approaches and determine whether in fact with input from outside stakeholders, whether these kinds of designs, this kind of way of developing drugs is going to produce the sort of good evidence, solid evidence that we need to make sure this product is safe and effective when it goes on the market.

Mr. Bucshon. OK, anything else? Well, anyone, for all of you, can anyone give us a sense of how they envision the FDA utilizing the authorities in 21st Century Cures Act in PDUFA VI, that the provisions involving the use of real-world, so-called real-world evidence to support their decision making how we would envision that being incorporated?

Ms. Holcombe. Well, I think as Dr. Woodcock said, FDA already uses real-world evidence in the determination, making determinations about potential safety signals of marketed drugs. So the question is in PDUFA VI, is it possible to use real-world evidence, i.e., patient experience with drugs in the marketplace from medical records or from your Apple watch? Is it possible to harness those data, to validate those data, and to use those data to understand more about how the drug is working, and would those data be helpful then in making a decision about perhaps broadening an indication for a drug that is very narrowly indicated or adding an indication, which goes to the point that Dr. Allen was making about how the drug label can become out of date when medical practice is ahead of what was known at the time the drug was produced.

Mr. Bucshon. OK. I will just make a quick comment. That is why other issues we are working on like interoperability of electronic medical records is going to be really key to this type of thing. I think everyone would agree to that and I yield back.

Mr. Guthrie. The gentleman yields back. Seeing no questions from this side, Ms. Brooks from Indiana is recognized for 5 minutes for purpose of asking questions.

Mrs. Brooks. Thank you, Mr. Chairman.

Dr. Pritchett, PDUFA VI creates a significantly revised fee structure which replaces current levies on manufacturing facilities and on products. Can you explain this revised fee structure and how is it beneficial for all parties?

Ms. Pritchett. I would actually yield to Kay who was directly involved in the negotiations and I wasn't, who I think would be better.

Mrs. Brooks. I wondered about that after one of her previous answers, but I was suggested to you. So Ms. Holcombe, would you like to share with us?

Ms. Holcombe. The reason for looking at a different way of collecting fees was to try to make sure that we had a system that was administratively as simple as it could be so that it was not so costly or so burdensome on either the FDA and companies. So the way fees used to be collected was they were divided one third among manufacturing facility fees, product fees, and application fees. There were two things wrong with that, at least two.

One thing was that it placed equal emphasis in terms of percentage of dollars collected on all three components, including the application fee which is the least predictable source of revenue. There is very little perfect ability to predict the number of applications that are going to come into FDA on an annual basis. They have a lot of experience so they can give you a range, but if you collect 50 instead of 60 that makes a huge difference in the total revenue that you are collecting. So could we reduce the dependence on the application fee and increase the dependence on other fees?

The second thing that was wrong was the manufacturing facility fee, which is a nightmare to calculate mostly because drugs aren't just manufactured like I make mine in my facility and you make yours in your facility. Lots of people make drugs in the same facility, so figuring out whose was where when and how often and so forth. So could we offload that fee, could we calculate the rest of the fee based on number of products?

And so we calculated what would that mean if we did certain percentages of collection from that new fee and certain percentage from the application fee? And we developed, or FDA actually developed, not I personally, a tool that companies could use and they could plug into this tool how much money they had paid in fees in previous years and how much they would pay under some new sort of split of the fees.

Mrs. Brooks. What is the tool referred to by the FDA?

Ms. Holcombe. We called it a widget, OK.

Mrs. Brooks. OK.

Ms. Holcombe. Yes, my terminology, sorry. It was a tool that allowed you to manipulate the percentage based on, so the total fee collection, let's say, is $800 million. If you collected ten percent from applications and 90 percent from products, what would that mean for each company? How much would they pay?

So they would plug in their own numbers, like how many applications did they think they would be submitting next year and how many products do they have on the market? And they figured out, bingo, up came this number; this is how much you pay. Well, then they could change that from 10/90 to 20/80. How much would you pay based on your number of products on the market and the number of applications you anticipate submitting, how much would you pay?

And using that tool, we figured out collectively with all of our companies that the ratio that had the least negative impact on the most companies was a 20 percent application fee, 80 percent program fee collection. And although a small number of companies on a percentage basis, out of all the long list of companies that pay fees, did see that their fees would go up slightly, the vast majority of companies saw that their fees actually would go down.

How could that even be, right, but it was. I mean, math, it is just a wonderful science.

Mrs. Brooks. And if those fees go down what happens?

Ms. Holcombe. The total amount of money collected is still the same because it is spread out across all fee payers.

Mrs. Brooks. OK, thank you. I am sorry my time is up, but thank you for explaining it.

Ms. Holcombe. I am sorry I don't know the math involved in it.

Mrs. Brooks. I yield back. OK, thank you.

Mr. Guthrie. Thank you, and the gentlelady yields back. Mr. Bilirakis is recognized for 5 minutes for questions.

Mr. Bilirakis. Thank you. Thank you, Mr. Chairman. I appreciate it very much.

Ms. Holcombe, back in the 2000s it was recognized that there was a lack of good information on the safety and efficacy of drugs for the pediatric population. Can you talk about some of the incentives that came about to encourage more pediatric clinical studies?

Ms. Holcombe. So the Best Pharmaceuticals for Children Act combined with the Pediatric Research Equity Act have been a very successful way to get more drugs studied in pediatric populations so that information can go on the drug label and pediatricians know how to dose the drugs for children. The incentive that has caused that to be so successful was the addition to whatever regulatory exclusivity the company might have on its product for adults of 6 months for doing these pediatric studies.

And we believe at BIO that incentives such as this one can be very effective in increasing the number of products that are developed in areas for which there is high unmet medical need but very difficult populations or areas of interest, such as, for example, intractable antibacterial resistant conditions. These are tough and there is just no good way of doing it. So incentives can be very effective and they have been for pediatric studies.

Mr. Bilirakis. What about the rare disease space? Again there are about 500 approved rare disease drugs, but 7,000 rare diseases affecting approximately 30 million Americans. They are taking medication off-label, and I know the stories because I hear from my constituents on a regular basis. They take the drugs off-label not knowing if their drugs are safe and effective for their conditions or if it is proper dosage—that is so important—and fighting with their insurance companies on coverage of these medications.

Does it make sense to incentivize development for a targeted population when there are clearly defined needs?

Ms. Holcombe. Yes.

Mr. Bilirakis. Thank you. Last month my colleague and I, G.K. Butterfield, introduced the OPEN Act for the second time. Much like the BPCA, it creates an incentive to run more clinical trials in the rare disease space where 95 percent of diseases have no FDA approval treatments. This would bring more approved drugs to these patients.

The OPEN Act has the potential to result in hundreds of new drugs and treatments for individuals with rare diseases. Only 150 rare disease patient groups, over 150 at last count, I think it is more than that support this bill. The OPEN Act was part of the House 21st Century Cures Act, and while it fell out at the 11th hour, unfortunately, I am going to continue to push for this legislation. It is a priority for me. Do you have any comments on that? And of course I welcome cosponsors for this legislation as well.

Ms. Holcombe. So it is clear that without the Orphan Drug Act we would not have 500 treatments for rare diseases. It is also a tragedy that we don't have 7,500. And again we believe incentives can work. We don't have an official position on your proposal, but definitely it merits more evaluation.

Mr. Bilirakis. All right. Well, thank you very much. I yield back, Mr. Chairman.

Mr. Guthrie. Thank you. The gentleman yields back, and seeing no other members wishing to ask questions I would like to thank all of our witnesses for being here today.

And pursuant to committee rules I remind members that they have 10 business days to submit additional questions for the record, and I ask the witnesses submit their response within 10 business days upon receipt of those questions.

Without objection, the subcommittee is adjourned.

[Whereupon, at 12:18 p.m., the subcommittee was adjourned.]

[Material submitted for inclusion in the record follows:]

PREPARED STATEMENT OF HON. FRANK PALLONE, JR.

Thank you, Mr. Chairman. I appreciate the opportunity today to discuss the reauthorization of the Prescription Drug User Fee Act. PDUFA has been incredibly successful at bringing reviews of new drug applications down by more than half, and providing patient access to treatments more quickly, and often before any other country.

PDUFA has also encouraged innovation by bringing stability and predictability to the review of new drug applications. FDA has been able to hire the review staff and scientific and technical experts needed to keep pace with science and increase the efficiency of the review process. However, more work needs to be done and I am encouraged by how PDUFA VI builds off of the successes of this user fee program.

I am therefore disappointed to see what can only be referred to as a disclaimer in the testimony today from FDA. While it is true that the reauthorization proposals were negotiated under a previous Administration, the goals of the PDUFA program and the drug approval process remain the same – a fully resourced and staffed FDA, and an efficient and timely drug review process that is keeping pace with the scientific and regulatory advancements in this field. It is my hope that the Administration would understand how carefully crafted the current agreement is, and recognize that the reauthorization process started nearly two years ago.

The agreement before us today is the result of many negotiations with industry and stakeholders, consultations with patients and consumers, and solicitation of public input. The resulting recommendations were transmitted to Congress in meeting the January 15, 2017 statutory deadline. Transmitting new recommendations at this point would go against this requirement, and run the very real risk of PDUFA not being reauthorized before the program expires on September 30, endangering the review of innovative new drug treatments and threatening the jobs of thousands of FDA employees.

I intend to continue to work with my colleagues on the Committee and across the Capitol, as well as industry, to ensure that we do not let this happen. This is a strong agreement, and one that deserves our support.

Thank you.

Rare Disease Legislative Advocates

Congress Begins Process of Reauthorizing Prescription Drug User Fee Act

March 16, 2017

Timely reauthorization of the Prescription Drug User Fee Act (PDUFA) was one of the hot issues discussed during the Legislative Conference during Rare Disease Week on Capitol Hill.

First enacted in 1992, PDUFA enables the Food and Drug Administration (FDA) to collect user fees from biopharmaceutical companies in order to enable the Agency to review the safety and efficacy of new medicines more quickly. According to PhRMA, it took FDA more than two years to review new medicines and more than 70% of medicines were approved outside of the U.S. before PDUFA.

Every five years, FDA and the biopharmaceutical industry negotiate a new user fee agreement, which Congress must enact in legislation. PDUFA was reauthorized in 2012 in the Food and Drug Administration Safety and

Innovation Act, which also included provisions creating the Breakthrough Therapy designation as well as the Rare Pediatric Disease Priority Voucher program. PDUFA is due to be reauthorized this year, as the current user fee agreement expires on September 30th.

Released last year, the draft PDUFA VI agreement includes specific performance goals for drug review, proposed plans for enhanced use of biomarkers, expanded patient engagement, and improved specialization of reviewers for rare diseases.

The Senate Health, Education, Labor and Pensions Committee will convene a hearing on PDUFA reauthorization on March 21st at 10am ET with testimony from senior FDA leadership, and will be available by livestream. The House Energy and Commerce Subcommittee on Health will hold a hearing on PDUFA on March 22nd at 10:15am.

As discussed on the March webinar, it is important for PDUFA to be reauthorized by the end of July or FDA will need to send furlough notices to staff who review new medicines.

http://rareadvocates.org/congress-begins-process-of-reauthorizing-prescription-drug-user-fee- act/

EPILEPSY FOUNDATION

March 21, 2017

The Honorable Michael Burgess, Chairman
U.S. House of Representatives
Energy and Commerce Committee, Subcommittee on Health

The Honorable Gene Green, Ranking Member
U.S. House of Representatives
Energy and Commerce Committee, Subcommittee on Health

Dear Chairman Burgess & Ranking Member Green:

The Epilepsy Foundation strongly supports the reauthorization of the Food and Drug Administration's (FDA) user fee programs and commends the Energy and Commerce Subcommittee on Health for moving the PDUFA agreement forward in the subcommittee. The Epilepsy Foundation is committed to accelerating the development and approval of new therapies, especially to benefit those in our community with difficult to control seizures and those who experience significant side effects from existing therapies. We support a strong FDA that is responsive to the needs of the patient community and the innovations of scientific research and health care delivery. We urge Congress to move judiciously through the process of reauthorizing the user fee programs and to honor the negotiations that led to the agreements.

The Epilepsy Foundation is the leading national voluntary health organization that speaks on behalf of more than 3 million Americans with epilepsy and seizures. We foster the wellbeing of children and adults affected by seizures through research programs, educational activities, advocacy, and direct services. Epilepsy is a medical condition that produces seizures affecting a variety of mental and physical functions.

The ability of the FDA to properly evaluate and approve therapies so they can enter the market in a timely manner is critically important to the Epilepsy Foundation because of our interest in and need for medical innovation. While many significant advances have been made in epilepsy over the past several years, including the development of innovative medications, medical devices, and surgical options, unfortunately, the number of people with epilepsy who are still experiencing seizures, despite being treated for the condition, has not changed. Today, 1 in 26 Americans will develop epilepsy in their lifetime; however, there is no cure, and even with many drugs and treatment options, one third of people with epilepsy live with uncontrollable seizures. Uncontrolled seizures can lead to disability, injury, and even death. Innovation is of importance to the people with epilepsy for whom available treatments do not work, as well as all Americans living with complex chronic and rare conditions that are not appropriately managed with current treatment options.

These user fee agreements are the result of many years of discussion with all relevant stakeholders, including the FDA, industry, and the patient community. The policies and goals included in the agreements reflect what these stakeholders value and will help ensure advancements and improvements within the FDA and ultimately health care more broadly.

The Epilepsy Foundation applauds congressional and agency leadership for this agreement that will continue the trajectory of patient-centered innovation at the FDA.

Sincerely,

Philip M. Gattone
President & CEO
Epilepsy Foundation

Timely Reauthorization of PDUFA & MDUFA is Critical to VC-backed Life Science Breakthroughs

March 20th, 2017 by Charlotte Savercool & filed under Medical Innovation, NVCA Blog.

Thirty years ago, the median time for the Food and Drug Administration (FDA) approval of a new drug was 33 months. As one can imagine, major backlog at the agency caused significant delay to the approval and entry of potentially life-saving drugs in the market. To address this problem, Congress passed the Prescription Drug User Fee Act in 1992 to authorize the FDA to collect fees when new drug applications were submitted. Those user fees, paid for by the biopharmaceutical industry, supplemented Congressional funding for the agency to review new drug applications in a more timely and efficient manner. Ten years later, Congress passed the Medical Device User Fee and Modernization Act (MDUFA) after the FDA's medical device program experienced a substantial loss in resources, seeking to accomplish a shared goal (between industry and the FDA) of improving the review process for new medical devices.

Collectively referred to as the "UFAs", PDUFA and MDUFA must be reauthorized by Congress every five years. The reauthorization cycle prompts an important collaboration between the FDA and both biopharmaceutical and medical device industries on a number of items, including evaluation of FDA performance, establishing new goals and objectives, and the negotiation of user fees paid for by industry. Congress then receives the proposed user fee agreement from FDA to convene discussion hearings and ultimately to consider reauthorization legislation.

Life science investors are familiar with the FDA approval process for drugs and devices, and understand the need for a capable regulatory body to accelerate the medical innovation occurring within the industry. Venture investment has driven significant growth into many of our country's most innovative and lifesaving medical products. In fact, the number of life science deals accounted for 12.5% of the overall venture deal count in 2016, investing in some of the most transformative and promising advancements in health care. Last year, $7.79 billion of venture capital was invested in the pharmaceutical and biotechnology sector and $3.86 billion of venture capital was invested in healthcare devices and supplies, representing 17% of overall venture activity. Noteworthy examples of venture-backed life science companies include Moderna, a developer of drugs for genetic disorders, hemophilic and blood factors, and oncology; Human Longevity, a developer of genomics and cell therapy-based diagnostic and therapeutic technology; and CVRx, a developer of implantable technology for the treatment of high blood pressure and heart failure.

It is certainly true that many venture-backed life science startups have seen extraordinary success, but it is important to recognize that medical breakthroughs are extremely challenging and expensive to develop. Those breakthroughs are made even more challenging when there is a lack of certainty on whether FDA will properly staffed and funded. Providing stable funding and resources to meet performance standards at the FDA is absolutely essential for attracting future investment and further expanding our nation's vibrant medical innovation ecosystem.

Over the next several weeks, Members of the Senate HELP Committee and the House Energy and Commerce Committee will hold hearings to examine these user fee programs, starting first with PDUFA and moving to MDUFA later in the month. The UFAs are set to expire the end of September and we are encouraged that Congress is taking significant action toward reauthorization. At the same time, a packed legislative agenda means that Congress and the Trump Administration will need to prioritize reauthorization of the UFAs to meet the September 30 deadline. We encourage policymakers to work in a collaborative manner to ensure medical innovation continues unimpeded.

http://nvca.org/blog/timely-reauthorization-pdufa-mdufa-critical-vc-backed-life-science-breakthroughs/

NORD and Friends of Cancer Research Issue Joint Statement In Advance of This Week's Congressional Hearings on FDA User Fees

March 21, 2017. Washington, D.C., March 21, 2017—The National Organization for Rare Disorders (NORD) and Friends of Cancer Research, two leading organizations that collectively represent millions of Americans with cancer and rare diseases, issued the following statement in advance of this week's congressional hearings on the reauthorization of FDA user fees:

"We wish to congratulate the Senate Committee on Health, Education, Labor, and Pensions (HELP) and the House Committee on Energy and Commerce (E&C) for moving forward with the reauthorization of the FDA user fees. This week's hearings represent important steps forward in the renewal of these critical programs.

We also wish to convey our support for the Commitment letters already negotiated and finalized by FDA and regulated industries. The PDUFA Commitment Goals Letter includes several important improvements and advancements to FDA processes and initiatives. These include the continuance of the Patient-Focused Drug Development program, the strengthening of the Breakthrough expedited review pathway, and the expansion of the Rare Diseases program, among others.

The MDUFA Commitment Goals letter also contains several crucial reforms including the further inclusion of patient preference information and patient-reported outcomes in device development and review, as well as the creation of the National Evaluation System for health Technology (NEST).

Our request of the Committees of Jurisdiction and Congress as a whole is simple: please keep the user fee reauthorization process non-partisan, uncontentious, and focused on the patients FDA serves every day.

The FDA largely relies on user fees authorized by Congress to operate. Without the user fees, a majority of drug, biologic, and device reviewers would be laid off, and the necessary review of innovative therapies would be substantially impaired if not halted all together.

The user fee acts are far too important to jeopardize with controversial partisan policy topics. We recognize the desire for additional reforms related to therapeutic development incentives, review, and access. But we respectfully request that attempts to reform these areas without full bipartisan support are not pursued as part of the UFA reauthorizations.

The cancer and rare disease patient communities rely on FDA to ensure that innovative, safe, and effective treatments reach those in need. We thank the HELP and E&C Committees for moving forward with these critical funding mechanisms, and look forward to their swift and unimpeded passage."

https://www.focr.org/news/nord-and-friends-cancer-research-issue-joint-statement- advance-week%E2%80%99s-congressional-hearings

In: Prescription Drugs
Editor: Karen Sue McKinney
ISBN: 978-1-53617-288-1

Chapter 2

PRESCRIPTION DRUG MONITORING PROGRAMS (UPDATED)*

Lisa N. Sacco, Amanda K. Sarata and Johnathan H. Duff

ABSTRACT

In the midst of national concern over the opioid epidemic, federal and state officials are paying greater attention to the manner in which opioids are prescribed. Nearly all prescription drugs involved in overdoses are originally prescribed by a physician (rather than, for example, being stolen from pharmacies). Thus, attention has been directed toward better understanding how opioids are being prescribed and preventing the diversion of prescription drugs after the prescriptions are dispensed.

Prescription drug monitoring programs (PDMPs) maintain statewide electronic databases of prescriptions dispensed for controlled substances (i.e., prescription drugs with a potential for abuse that are subject to stricter government regulation). Information collected by PDMPs may be used to educate and inform prescribers, pharmacists, and the public; identify or prevent drug abuse and diversion; facilitate the identification of prescription drug-addicted individuals and enable intervention and

* This is an edited, reformatted and augmented version of Congressional Research Service, Publication No. R42593, dated May 24, 2018.

treatment; outline drug use and abuse trends to inform public health initiatives; or educate individuals about prescription drug use, abuse, diversion, and PDMPs themselves.

As of February 2018, 50 states, the District of Columbia, and two territories (Guam and Puerto Rico) had operational PDMPs within their borders.

How PDMPs are organized and operated varies among states. Each state determines which agency houses the PDMP; which controlled substances must be reported; which types of dispensers (e.g., pharmacies) are required to submit data; how often data are collected; who may access information in the PDMP database (e.g., prescribers, dispensers, or law enforcement); the circumstances under which the information may (or must) be accessed; and what enforcement mechanisms are in place for noncompliance.

PDMP costs may vary widely, with startup costs that can range as high as $450,000 to over $1.5 million and annual operating costs ranging from $125,000 to nearly $1.0 million. States finance PDMPs using monies from a variety of sources including the state general fund, prescriber and pharmacy licensing fees, state controlled substance registration fees, health insurers' fees, direct- support organizations, state grants, and/or federal grants.

The federal government supports state PDMPs through programs at the Departments of Justice (DOJ) and Health and Human Services (HHS). Since FY2002, DOJ has administered the Harold Rogers Prescription Drug Monitoring Program, and in FY2017, DOJ incorporated this grant program into the new Comprehensive Opioid Abuse Program. HHS programs include National All Schedules Prescription Electronic Reporting (NASPER), State Demonstration Grants for Comprehensive Opioid Abuse Response, Opioid Prevention in States grants, State Targeted Response to the Opioid Crisis Grants, and various pilots and initiatives under the Office of the National Coordinator for Health Information Technology (ONC). Of note, NASPER last received appropriations (of $2.0 million) in FY2010.

State PDMPs vary with respect to whether or how information contained in the database is shared with other states. Federal policymakers have repeatedly emphasized the importance of enhancing interstate information sharing and the interoperability of state PDMPs. In 2011, the Obama Administration included efforts to increase interstate data sharing in its action plan to counter prescription drug abuse. In 2017, a presidential commission recommended, among other things, that the Trump Administration support legislation to require DOJ to fund a "data-sharing hub" and require states receiving federal grant funds to share PDMP data.

The available evidence suggests that PDMPs can be effective in reducing the time required for drug diversion investigations, changing prescribing behavior, reducing "doctor shopping," and reducing prescription drug abuse. Assessments of effectiveness should also take into consideration potential unintended consequences of PDMPs, such as limiting access to medications for legitimate use or pushing drug diversion activities over the border into a neighboring state. Experts suggest that PDMP effectiveness might be improved by increasing the timeliness, completeness, consistency, and accessibility of the data.

Policy issues that might come before Congress include the role of state PDMPs in federal efforts to combat prescription drug abuse, the role of the federal government in interstate data-sharing and interoperability, and the possible link between the crackdown on prescription drug abuse and the uptick in illicit opioid (e.g., heroin and illicit fentanyl) abuse. While establishment and enhancement of PDMPs enjoy relatively broad support, stakeholders express concerns about health care versus law enforcement uses of PDMP data (particularly with regard to protection of personally identifiable health information).

INTRODUCTION

In the midst of national concern over the opioid epidemic and the large number of prescription opioid overdose deaths in the United States, federal and state officials are paying greater attention to the manner in which opioids are prescribed.[1] Prescription opioid-related overdose deaths dramatically increased from 1999 to 2010 in the United States in conjunction with increased opioid prescribing, and overdose deaths involving prescription opioids were five times higher in 2016 than in

[1] Centers for Disease Control and Prevention, *Understanding the Epidemic*, August 2017, http://www.cdc.gov/ drugoverdose/epidemic/index.html; The President's Commission on Combating Drug Addiction and the Opioid Crisis, *Final Report*, November 1, 2017, https://www.whitehouse.gov/sites/whitehouse.gov/files/images/ Final_Report_Draft_11-1-2017.pdf; and The White House, *FACT SHEET: Obama Administration Announces Public and Private Sector Efforts to Address Prescription Drug Abuse and Heroin Use*, https://obamawhitehouse.archives.gov/the-press-office/2015/10/21/fact-sheet-obama-administration-announces-public- and-private-sector (hereinafter, *FACT SHEET: Obama Administration Announces Public and Private Sector Efforts to Address Prescription Drug Abuse and Heroin Use*). Prescription drugs of abuse are often divided into the categories of *pain relievers* (e.g., oxycodone), central nervous system *stimulants* (e.g., amphetamine), and central nervous system *depressants* (e.g., benzodiazepines). Pain relievers that are subject to abuse may be called *narcotics* or *opioids*. Central nervous system depressants may be further divided into *tranquilizers* (also called *anxiolytics*, used to reduce anxiety) and *sedatives* (also called *sedative-hypnotics*, used to induce sleep). The term *psychotherapeutics* is sometimes used to capture all of these categories.

1999.[2] Over the last year, the Trump Administration, Congress, state governments, and the private sector have all taken action to address prescription drug abuse. Initiatives range from state and private health care initiatives, such as limiting the number of pills in a prescription, to major legislation, such as the Comprehensive Addiction and Recovery Act (CARA; P.L. 114- 198), which included many provisions to address prescription drug abuse.[3]

In 2016, an estimated 11.8 million individuals aged 12 or older (4.4% of this population) misused[4] opioids in the past year, including 11.5 million pain reliever misusers and 948,000 heroin users.[5] Prescription painkillers—natural and semisynthetic opioids (e.g., oxycodone, hydrocodone, and morphine) are involved in more overdose deaths than any other opioid.[6]

---

[2] Gera P. Guy Jr., Kun Zhang, Michele K. Bohm et al., Centers for Disease Control and Prevention (CDC), *Vital Signs: Changes in Opioid Prescribing in the United States, 2006-2015*, Morbidity and Mortality Weekly Report (MMWR), July 7, 2017, https://www.cdc.gov/mmwr/volumes/66/wr/mm6626a4.htm; and CDC, *Prescription Opioid Overdose Data*, https://www.cdc.gov/drugoverdose/data/overdose.html.

[3] CVSHealth, "CVS Health Fighting National Opioid Abuse Epidemic With Enterprise Initiatives," press release, September 21, 2017, https://cvshealth.com/newsroom/press-releases/cvs-health-fighting-national-opioid-abuse- epidemic-with-enterprise-initiatives; CVS Caremark, *CVS Caremark® Opioid Quantity Limits Pharmacy Reference Guide*, 2018, https://www.caremark.com/portal/asset/Opioid_Reference_Guide.pdf; Walmart, *Walmart Introduces Additional Measures to Help Curb Opioid Abuse and Misuse*, May 7, 2018, https://news.walmart.com/2018/05/07/ walmart-introduces-additional-measures-to-help-curb-opioid-abuse-and-misuse; and the Comprehensive Addiction and Recovery Act of 2016 (CARA; P.L. 114-198). For a review of state initiatives, see National Conference of State Legislatures, *Prevention of Prescription Drug Overdose and Abuse*, May 23, 2016, http://www.ncsl.org/research/health/prevention-of-prescription-drug-overdose-and-abuse.aspx.

[4] The National Survey on Drug Use and Mental Health (NSDUH) defines *misuse* as use in any way not directed by a doctor, including use without a prescription of one's own; use in greater amounts, more often, or longer than told to take a drug; or use in any other way not directed by a doctor. Misuse of over-the-counter drugs is not included. Terms such as *misuse*, *abuse*, *dependence*, and *addiction* are often used interchangeably with nonmedical use, although each term may have its own definition within a specific context.

[5] Some reported use of both heroin and pain relievers, so the numbers will not total to 11.5 million. U.S. Department of Health and Human Services, Substance Abuse and Mental Health Services Administration, *Results from the 2016 National Survey on Drug Use and Health: Summary of National Findings*, September 2017, https://www.samhsa.gov/data/sites/default/files/NSDUH-FFR1-2016/NSDUH-FFR1-2016.htm (hereinafter: *2016 National Survey on Drug Use and Health*).

[6] Rose A. Rudd, Noah Aleshire, and Jon E. Zibbell et al., Centers for Disease Control and Prevention, *Increases in Drug and Opioid Overdose Deaths—United States, 2000-2014*, Morbidity and Mortality Weekly Report (MMWR), January 1, 2016, http://www.cdc.gov/mmwr/preview/mmwrhtml/mm6450a3.htm.

Of the individuals who used prescription painkillers non-medically in 2016, more than half (53.0%) received the drugs from a friend or relative either for free, by purchase, or by stealing.[7] Aside from prescription painkillers such as oxycodone, other commonly abused prescription medications include benzodiazepines and amphetamine-like drugs.

Some academic and government experts link the crackdown on prescription drug abuse and the comparatively higher cost of prescription pain relievers on the black market to the uptick in heroin abuse.[8] The number of individuals aged 12 or older currently[9] using heroin (475,000 in 2016) has nearly tripled since 2002.[10] Like many prescription pain relievers, heroin is an opioid. Unlike prescription pain relievers, however, heroin is a Schedule I controlled substance under the Controlled Substances Act[11] and has no accepted medical use in the United States.

Most prescription drugs that are misused are *originally* prescribed by a physician (rather than, for example, being stolen from pharmacies); therefore, attention has been directed toward preventing the diversion of prescription drugs after the prescriptions are dispensed. Prescription drug monitoring programs (PDMPs) maintain statewide electronic databases of dispensed prescriptions for controlled substances. PDMP information can aid medical professionals and those in law enforcement in identifying

---

[7] *2016 National Survey on Drug Use and Health*, Figure 34, https://www.samhsa.gov/data/sites/default/files/NSDUH-FFR1-2016/NSDUH-FFR1-2016.htm.

[8] Pradip K. Muhuri, Joseph C. Gfroerer, and M. Christine Davies, *Associations of Nonmedical Pain Reliever Use and Initiation of Heroin Use in the United States*, Substance Abuse and Mental Health Services Administration, Center for Behavioral Health Statistics and Quality, August 2013, http://www.samhsa.gov/data/2k13/DataReview/DR006/ nonmedical-pain-reliever-use-2013.pdf; Theodore J. Cicero, Matthew S. Ellis, and Hilary L. Surratt, "Effect of Abuse- Deterrent Formulation of Oxycontin," *New England Journal of Medicine*, vol. 367, no. 2 (July 12, 2012), pp. 187-189;

U.S. Department of Justice, National Drug Intelligence Center, *National Drug Threat Assessment 2003*, "Narcotics", January 2003, http://www.justice.gov/archive/ndic/pubs3/3300/pharm.htm; and U.S. Department of Justice, National Drug Intelligence Center, *National Drug Threat Assessment 2011*, August 2011, p. 37, http://www.justice.gov/archive/ ndic/pubs44/44849/44849p.pdf.

[9] NSDUH defines "current" use as any use in the past 30 days.

[10] *Results from the 2016 National Survey on Drug Use and Health*.

[11] 21 U.S.C. §801 et seq.

patterns of prescribing, dispensing, or receiving controlled substances that may indicate abuse.[12]

For over a decade, the federal government has provided financial support for state-level PDMPs. In 2002, Congress established the Harold Rogers PDMP grant, administered by the Department of Justice (DOJ), to help law enforcement, regulatory entities, and public health officials analyze data on prescriptions for controlled substances. Three years later, Congress and the President enacted the National All Schedules Prescription Electronic Reporting Act of 2005 (NASPER) requiring the Secretary of Health and Human Services (HHS) to award grants to states to establish or improve PDMPs. In 2016, CARA authorized PDMP activity under two grant programs administered by DOJ and HHS.

Congress has demonstrated a particular interest in facilitating interoperability among state-level PDMPs, as well as in establishing national programs.[13] Policymakers have focused on enhancing state-level databases and interstate information sharing, and some have suggested establishing a national system. Related issues that policymakers may consider are whether PDMPs and their interstate information-sharing platforms adequately protect personally identifiable and related health information, and whether they can ensure that patients with legitimate medical needs have access to prescriptions. Congress may also exercise oversight with respect to the role of PDMPs in the Administration's efforts to combat the prescription drug epidemic;[14] policymakers may assess the extent to which the relevant departments and agencies have taken steps to accomplish these PDMP-related goals.

---

[12] Initiatives countering prescription drug abuse range from prevention and treatment to enforcement. These activities include scheduling chemicals used in certain prescription drugs, supporting public awareness campaigns, bolstering law enforcement, and providing assistance to states—in part through PDMPs. This chapter focuses on PDMPs.

[13] These issues were addressed in Section 1141 of the Food and Drug Administration Safety and Innovation Act (P.L. 112-144).

[14] The President's Commission on Combating Drug Addiction and the Opioid Crisis, *Final Report*, November 1, 2017, https://www.whitehouse.gov/sites/whitehouse.gov/files/images/Final_Report_Draft_11-1-2017.pdf; and *FACT SHEET: Obama Administration Announces Public and Private Sector Efforts to Address Prescription Drug Abuse and Heroin Use*.

This chapter provides an overview of PDMPs, including their operation, enforcement mechanisms, costs, and financing. It also examines the effectiveness of PDMPs and outlines federal grants supporting PDMPs. Finally, this chapter discusses relevant considerations for policymakers including interstate data sharing, interoperability, protection of health information, and the possible link between the crackdown on prescription drug abuse and rise in heroin abuse.

PRESCRIPTION DRUG MONITORING PROGRAMS (PDMPS)

PDMPs maintain statewide electronic databases of designated information on specified prescription drugs dispensed within the states. Data are made available to individuals or organizations as authorized under state law; these may include prescribers, law enforcement officials, licensing boards, or others. Possible uses of PDMPs include

- identifying or preventing drug abuse and diversion;
- facilitating the identification of prescription drug-addicted individuals and appropriate intervention and treatment;
- outlining use and abuse trends to inform public health initiatives; and
- educating individuals about prescription drug use, abuse, and diversion.[15]

In addition to uses of PDMPs aimed at drug abuse and diversion, an explicit goal of PDMPs is supporting access to controlled substances for legitimate medical use. This may best be understood by viewing PDMPs in comparison to earlier, paper-based programs called multiple- copy prescription programs. For example, in 1914 a New York state law required physicians to use state-issued, serialized, duplicate prescription

---

[15] The Prescription Drug Monitoring Program Training and Technical Assistance Center, *The Goals of Prescription Monitoring*; National Alliance for Model State Drug Laws, *Prescription Drug Monitoring Programs: A Brief Overview*, August 17, 2010.

forms for certain drugs.[16] Similarly, California began a multiple-copy prescription program using triplicate forms for specified narcotics in 1939; it expanded to monitor all schedule II narcotics in 1972 and schedule II non-narcotics in 1981.[17] Studies of multiple-copy prescription programs found that many prescribers did not order the required prescription forms, rendering them unable to prescribe specified controlled substances even when medically appropriate.[18] In addition, the ability to check a patient's prescription history using an electronic PDMP might give prescribers more confidence when considering the use of drugs with high risk of abuse and prevent the prescribing of contraindicated medications.

As of February 2018, 50 states, the District of Columbia, and two territories (Guam and Puerto Rico) had operational PDMPs within their borders.[19]

Program Operation

The entity responsible for administering the PDMP varies by state and may be a pharmacy board, department of health, professional licensing agency, law enforcement agency, substance abuse agency, or consumer protection agency. Of the authorized state PDMPs (including the District

---

[16] Scott M. Fishman et al., "Regulating Opioid Prescribing Through Prescription Monitoring Programs: Balancing Drug Diversion and Treatment of Pain," *Pain Medicine*, vol. 5, no. 3 (2004), pp. 309-324.

[17] Aaron M. Gilson et al., "Time Series Analysis of California's Prescription Monitoring Program: Impact on Prescribing and Multiple Provider Episodes," *Journal of Pain*, vol. 13, no. 2 (2012), pp. 103-111.

[18] Scott M. Fishman et al., "Regulating Opioid Prescribing Through Prescription Monitoring Programs: Balancing Drug Diversion and Treatment of Pain," *Pain Medicine*, vol. 5, no. 3 (2004), pp. 309-324.

[19] In July 2017, Missouri Governor Eric Greitens signed an executive order directing the Missouri Department of Health and Human Services to establish a PDMP. While St. Louis County, MO, already had an operational PDMP that incorporated other counties in Missouri, it is unclear if the *state* has an operational PDMP. CRS attempted to reach the Missouri Department of Health and Human Services to discuss this matter on January 31, 2018, but was referred to the St. Louis County PDMP.

of Columbia), most (40) are administered by either pharmacy boards or health departments.[20]

Schedules of Controlled Substances

The Controlled Substances Act (21 U.S.C. §801 et seq.) establishes schedules for controlled substances (including drugs), ranging from schedule I (most restrictive) to schedule V (least restrictive). Drugs on schedule I have no currently accepted medical use in the United States and are not available by prescription. Drugs with recognized medical uses are on schedules II through V, with each successive schedule representing a lower risk of abuse.

State laws determine which schedules of controlled substances are monitored under each program (see text box for a brief explanation of schedules), what information is to be submitted, the means by which dispensers or dispensaries submit the required information, and the time frame in which information must be submitted.

Each state also determines which entities dispensing prescriptions for controlled substances are required to submit data to the PDMP. Most states require retail pharmacies and dispensing practitioners (e.g., physicians and/or veterinarians) to submit data to the PDMP.[21] Some states also have statutory authority to require out-of-state, mail order, and Internet pharmacies to submit data to the PDMP regarding prescription or controlled drugs dispensed to residents of thestate.

For instance, if a patient in Alabama receives a prescription for a monitored drug from an out-of- state mail order pharmacy, the mail order pharmacy must report the prescription to the Alabama PDMP.[22]

Of note, information on medications (e.g., methadone or buprenorphine) dispensed at federally assisted drug treatment programs generally may not be reported to PDMPs without patient consent under

---

[20] Research current through June 30, 2017. National Alliance for Model State Drug Laws (NAMSDL), *Prescription Drug Monitoring Program (PMP) Administering Agency*, 2017, http://www.namsdl.org.

[21] NAMSDL, *Reporting Requirements and Exemptions to Reporting, Compilation of Statutes,* May 2016, http://www.namsdl.org/prescription-monitoring-programs.cfm.

[22] NAMSDL, *States With Statutory Authority to Require Nonresident Pharmacies to Report to Prescription Monitoring Program*, May 2016, http://www.namsdl.org/.

federal privacy regulations (42 C.F.R. Part 2). These regulations place strict limitations on the disclosure, and redisclosure, of patient information created and maintained by such programs that identifies the individual patient as a drug abuser, or links the individual to the program.[23]

Access to information contained in the PDMP database is determined by state law and varies by state. The majority of states allow pharmacists and practitioners to access information related to their patients, and some also allow other entities—law enforcement, licensing and regulatory boards, state Medicaid Programs, state medical examiners, and research organizations—to access the information under certain circumstances.[24] State laws outline the procedures by which information from the PDMP may be accessed.

With respect to how the states identify and investigate cases of potential prescription drug diversion or abuse, PDMPs may be classified as *reactive* or *proactive*. In essence, "[s]tates with [r]eactive PDMPs ... generate solicited reports only in response to a specific inquiry made by a prescriber, dispenser, or other party with appropriate authority" while "[s]tates with [p]roactive PDMPs ... identify and investigate cases, generating unsolicited reports whenever suspicious behavior is detected."[25]

Interstate Information Sharing and Interoperability

State PDMPs vary widely with respect to whether or how information contained in the database is shared with other states. While some states do not have measures in place allowing interstate sharing of information, others have specific policies that govern sharing of information across state lines. These policies may be based on factors such as agreed-upon

[23] See CRS In Focus IF10374, *Health Privacy: Updating Federal Protections for Patient Records at Substance Abuse Treatment Programs*.

[24] Researchers may be allowed de-identified data for analysis and research purposes. See PDMP Training and Technical Assistance Center, *Prescription Monitoring Frequently Asked Questions (FAQ)*, http://www.pdmpassist.org/ content/prescription-drug-monitoring-frequently-asked-questions-faq.

[25] Ronald Simeone and Lynn Holland, *Executive Summary: An Evaluation of Prescription Drug Monitoring Programs*, Simeone Associates, Inc., http://www.namsdl.org/.

reciprocity between states, or whether a request stems from an ongoing investigation.[26] As of September 20, 2017, 43 states were engaged in interstate data sharing while 5 states were still implementing interstate data sharing.[27]

Researchers provided states with guidance in creating memoranda of understanding (MOUs) for interstate data exchange. Questions that states may consider when drafting an MOU include the following:[28]

- How is the information to be reported?
- How will the information be used by the relevant states?
- What are the guidelines on data retention?
- What are the state responsibilities in the event of a data breach?
- Are there measures in place for conflict resolution?
- What are the consequences of potential data misuse?

In addition, the Council of State Governments highlighted four areas as central to the success of interstate compacts regarding PDMPs and data sharing:

> Education—responsibility of providers, data integrity, training requirements (start up versus ongoing)[;]
>
> Funding—state funding, costs of data sharing, costs of operation[;]
>
> Security and Access—authorized users, authentication, audit trails, Internet access, vendor security, reporting, privacy, confidentiality, use of data[; and]
>
> Technology—data transfer and exchange, uniformity and standards, cost reduction, compatibility, quality/error correction[.][29]

[26] National Alliance for Model State Drug Laws, *Interstate Sharing of Prescription Monitoring Database Information*, May 2016, http://www.namsdl.org.

[27] For a map depicting the interstate sharing of PDMP data, see http://www.pdmpassist.org/pdf/Interstate_Data_Sharing_20170920.pdf.

[28] Alliance of States With Prescription Monitoring Programs and Brandeis University's Training and Technical Assistance Center, *Memorandum Of Understanding: Writing Guide for States with Prescription Monitoring Programs*, funded through a grant (No. 2010-DG-BX-K088) from the Bureau of Justice Assistance.

[29] The Council of State Governments, National Center for Interstate Compacts, *Prescription Drug Monitoring Programs: Interstate Compact—National Advisory Panel*, November 5-6, 2009, http://www.csg.org/pubs/capitolideas/ enews/enewsissue38/21stCenturyHandout.pdf.

Without funding, data sharing, and knowledgeable users actively participating in PDMPs, these programs cannot be effective.

Efforts are ongoing to facilitate information sharing using prescription monitoring information exchange (PMIX) architecture—an information exchange standard/nationwide framework that applies to PDMP systems, data sharing "hubs", such as RxCheck,[30] and other exchange partners or intermediaries.[31] The PMIX program is intended to enable the interstate exchange of PDMP information, providing information on an individual's prescription drug history to states participating in the information exchange. This information can help identify potential prescription drug abuse or diversion, and can help inform stakeholders such as law enforcement, health and human services, health practitioners, and public regulatory agencies. A state can participate in the PMIX program if it has

- legislation allowing it to share patient information with other states in real time,
- identified at least one other state as a partner in the information exchange, and
- either (1) established an MOU with their identified partner(s) in the information exchange or (2) ratified the Prescription Monitoring Interstate Compact.[32]

The infrastructure of the PMIX program is based on the National Information Exchange Model (NIEM), which is a "common vocabulary"

[30] As of January 17, 2018, five states were actively using RxCheck as their interstate data sharing hub. Twelve additional states were either implementing interstate data sharing via RxCheck or planning to connect to RxCheck. See PDMP Training and Technical Assistance Center, *Interstate Data Sharing via RxCheck Hub*, http://www.pdmpassist.org/pdf/RxCheck_Hub_states_20180117.pdf.

[31] More information on PMIX can be found at http://www.pdmpassist.org and http://www.ijis.org. A pilot project between Kentucky and Ohio's PDMPs formed the springboard for the larger PMIX initiative. Through this pilot, a PMIX hub server was installed in Ohio, and Ohio and Kentucky signed an MOU for data exchange, see IJIS Institute, *Cross-Boundary Initiatives*, http://www.ijis.org.

[32] *Prescription Monitoring Information Exchange (PMIX) Architecture*, Brandeis University, Prescription Drug Monitoring Program Training and Technical Assistance Center, http://www.pdmpassist.org/content/prescription-drug- monitoring-information-architecture-pmix.

used by the public and private sector to exchange information.[33] To facilitate information security and data privacy, data are encrypted while passing through "hubs," and no data are actually stored on these hubs. PMIX allows for hubs to exist at the state and national levels, and it allows for hub-to-hub information exchange.[34]

With pharmaceutical industry support, the National Association of Boards of Pharmacy (NABP) developed a technology platform to facilitate interstate sharing of PDMP data, called InterConnect, which NABP committed to make compliant with PMIX architecture.[35]

Although there are no federal requirements for state PDMP interoperability and information sharing, Congress and the President enacted legislation that

- authorized the HHS Secretary, consulting with the Attorney General as appropriate, to "facilitate … the development of recommendations on interoperability standards" for interstate information exchange by states receiving specified federal grants to support their PDMPs;
- required the HHS Secretary, in so doing, to consider the PMIX standards; and
- required the HHS Secretary to submit "a report on enhancing the interoperability of [state PDMPs] with other technologies and databases used for detecting and reducing fraud, diversion, and abuse of prescription drugs."[36]

---

[33] See the government website for the National Information Exchange Model (NIEM): https://www.niem.gov/.

[34] PDMP Training and Technical Assistance Center and Alliance of States With Prescription Monitoring Programs, *PMIX National Architecture Overview*, http://www.pdmpassist.org/pdf/ PMIX%20National%20Architecture%20Overview.pdf.

[35] U.S. Department of Justice, Office of Justice Programs, Bureau of Justice Assistance, BJA Policy on Use of Harold Rogers Prescription Drug Monitoring Program (HRPDMP) Funding to Support Interstate Data Sharing Activities, May 30, 2012, https://www.bja.gov/Programs/PDMPPolicy.pdf. This supersedes interim policy guidance documentation dated March 21, 2012, and April 17, 2012.

[36] Section 1141 of the Food and Drug Administration Safety and Innovation Act (P.L. 112-144).

In 2013, HHS submitted its report to Congress on PDMP interoperability standards. In addressing legal and policy challenges, HHS recommended that states ensure that PDMPs do not restrict access to PDMP data for health care providers and enact laws and policies to increase use of PDMPs by health care providers, among other recommendations.[37] In addressing interoperability and technology issues, HHS recommended that state PDMPs implement interoperability standards "that best support the information's use upon its exchange," among other recommendations.[38] HHS stressed the importance of unsolicited reports from PDMPs to providers, licensing boards, regulatory and law enforcement agencies, and public and private insurers and pharmacy benefit managers.[39] The report also reviews literature on PDMP effectiveness and health provider use of PDMPs.

Over the past several years, federal grant funds have gone toward improving interoperability and information sharing between states, and there are reports of successful initiation and expansion of interstate information sharing. For example, SAMHSA funded PDMP integration and interoperability projects in nine states from FY2012 to FY2016 and released a report outlining challenges and successes.[40]

Compliance and Enforcement Mechanisms

In ensuring that a given state's PDMP reflects comprehensive data from all relevant pharmacies, physicians, and other dispensaries, one principal concern is how to ensure that they are reporting prescription data to the program. The laws or rules governing consequences for failure to

---

[37] U.S. Department of Health and Human Services, *Prescription Drug Monitoring Program Interoperability Standards*, A Report to Congress, September 2013, http://www.healthit.gov/sites/default/files/fdasia1141report_final.pdf.

[38] Ibid., pp. 5, 21. For specific recommendations, see the full report.

[39] Ibid., pp. 4, 17-18.

[40] Centers for Disease Control and Prevention, National Center for Injury Prevention and Control, Division of Unintentional Injury Prevention, *Integrating & Expanding Prescription Drug Monitoring Program Data: Lessons from Nine States*, February 2017, https://www.cdc.gov/drugoverdose/pdf/pehriie_report-a.pdf.

report data are determined by each state. For example, one consequence may be disciplinary action by the appropriate licensing board or commission. Another may be that failure to report information could trigger the PDMP program office to report the lapse in compliance to the PDMP governing agency, which may then refer the information to law enforcement.[41]

Program Costs

PDMP expenses involve startup costs, funds needed to operate and maintain the programs, and any monies used to enhance program operation and interoperability. Overall program costs can entail

- hardware such as servers;
- software to run the PDMP database and ensure information security;
- connectivity such that pharmacies and dispensaries can enter data, and prescribers and/or law enforcement officials can request and access data;
- staff to administer the PDMP and provide technical assistance; and
- overhead fees.

A 2009 evaluation by the Maryland Advisory Council on Prescription Drug Monitoring assessed existing state PDMPs on a range of factors including the costs associated with establishing and maintaining the programs.[42] The overarching finding was that costs vary widely, with program startup costs ranging from $450,000 to over $1.5 million. Further,

[41] See, for example, Florida's PDMP rule states that "[t]he program will file a complaint with the Department and refer to law enforcement any failure to report the dispensing of Schedules II – IV controlled substances." Rule 64K-1.004, https://www.flrules.org/gateway/RuleNo.asp?title=Prescription%20Drug%20Monitoring%20Program&ID=64K-1.004.

[42] Maryland Advisory Council on Prescription Drug Monitoring, *Maryland Advisory Council on Prescription Drug Monitoring Legislative Report*, December 31, 2009, p. 76, http://msa.maryland.gov/megafile/msa/speccol/sc5300/sc5339/000113/012000/012478/unrestricted/20100355e.pdf.

based on available data from six operational PDMPs, the Maryland Advisory Council's evaluation indicates that annual operating costs range from $125,000 to nearly $1.0 million, with an average annual cost of about $500,000. The Maryland Advisory Council reported that

> [c]ost variations are affected by the frequency of data collection (e.g., daily, weekly, bi- weekly, monthly), the use of third party vendors for data collection and analysis, the number of prescriptions written and filled in the state, the number of drug schedules (II-V) and drugs of interest collected, and the use of official forms or other required collection and submission mechanisms.[43]

A 2002 Government Accountability Office (GAO) evaluation of PDMP costs in Kentucky, Nevada, and Utah revealed findings similar to those presented by the Maryland Advisory Council. GAO noted a number of PDMP design and operational factors driving variations in state costs for running PDMPs. Specifically, these involved "differences in the PDMP systems implemented, the number of pharmacies reporting drug dispensing data, and the number of practitioners and law enforcement agencies seeking information from the systems."[44]

PDMP Financing

States finance the startup and operation of PDMPs through a variety of channels. PDMP financing often involves monies from the state general fund, prescriber and pharmacy licensing fees, state controlled substance registration fees, health insurers' fees, direct-support organizations, state or

---

[43] Maryland Advisory Council on Prescription Drug Monitoring, *Maryland Advisory Council on Prescription Drug Monitoring Legislative Report*, December 31, 2009, pp. 76-77. An earlier (2002) evaluation of PDMPs by the Government Accountability Office (GAO) found similar reasons for variability in state costs for PDMP operation. These variations were driven by "differences in the PDMP systems implemented, the number of pharmacies reporting drug dispensing data, and the number of practitioners and law enforcement agencies seeking information from the systems."

[44] U.S. General Accounting Office, *Prescription Drugs: State Monitoring Programs Provide Useful Tool to Reduce Diversion*, GAO-02-634, May 2002, p. 3, http://www.gao.gov/assets/240/234687.pdf.

federal grants, or a combination thereof.[45] Guidelines for how states may fund PDMPs are outlined in each state's PDMP authorizing legislation. For example, Oregon's PDMP has a fund within the state treasury. This fund receives monies, in part, from a proportion of medical provider fees. These fees are paid to the appropriate medical board, and the board in turn transmits a portion of these fees to the PDMP fund. The Oregon Department of Human Services, which administers the PDMP, may also accept and deposit into the fund money from a variety of additional sources, including grants and donations.[46]

Some states prohibit the use of certain sources of funding, thus limiting the potential range of funding mechanisms. For instance, Florida law specifically prohibits the use of state funds or funds received—directly or indirectly—from prescription drug manufacturers to support the PDMP.[47] As such, the program receives funding from three sources: the Florida PDMP Foundation, Inc., an organization established in Florida law for the purpose of funding the PDMP; federal grants; and private grants.[48]

PDMP EFFECTIVENESS

The available evidence suggests that PDMPs are effective in some ways for both law enforcement and health care purposes; however, research on the effectiveness of PDMPs is limited, especially in the area of law enforcement. Experts suggest that PDMPs have the potential to be more effective.

---

[45] Alliance of States With Prescription Monitoring Programs, *Prescription Monitoring Programs: Funding Mechanisms & Business Models*, National Legislation & Implementation Meeting 2010, 2010, p. 3, http://www.pdmpassist.org/pdf/PPTs/LI2010/PMP-FundingBus Models.pdf.

[46] Oregon PDMP statute (ORS 431.960 et seq.).

[47] Title XLVI, Section 893.055, Florida Statutes - Prescription Drug Monitoring Program.

[48] Florida Department of Health, *Funding the E-FORSCE Database*, http://www. floridahealth.gov/statistics-and-data/e- forcse/funding/index.html.

Effectiveness Research

Research on PDMP effectiveness suggests that they have an impact on both law enforcement and health care. A 2002 GAO study found that "the time and effort required by law enforcement and regulatory investigators to explore leads and the merits of possible drug diversion cases" declined after PDMP implementation.[49] The study found that investigations of alleged doctor shoppers by Kentucky officials took an average of 156 days prior to PDMP implementation and 16 days after PDMP implementation (a 90% decrease). Nevada and Utah also reported decreases in investigation time of 83% and 80%, respectively. It is important to note that decreases in investigation time do not necessarily translate into less prescription drug abuse.

A 2012 review article summarized all peer-reviewed research articles about PDMPs published between 2001 and 2011, which amounted to 11 articles (not all of which addressed effectiveness).[50] The author concluded that PDMPs reduce "doctor shopping," change prescribing behavior, and reduce prescription drug abuse. For example, a 2006 federally funded study (included in the 2012 review article) found that PDMPs—especially ones that issue reports proactively—change prescriber behavior in a way that reduces the per capita supply of prescription pain relievers and stimulants, which in turn reduces the likelihood of abuse.[51] Another study published in 2012 (and therefore not included in the review article) found

---

[49] U.S. General Accounting Office, *Prescription Drugs: State Monitoring Programs Provide Useful Tool to Reduce Diversion*, GAO-02-634, May 2002, p. 3, http://www.gao.gov/assets/240/234687.pdf.

[50] Julie Worley, "Prescription Drug Monitoring Programs, a Response to Doctor Shopping: Purpose, Effectiveness, and Directions for Future Research," *Issues in Mental Health Nursing*, vol. 33, no. 5 (2012), pp. 319-328. Note: The GAO study was not included, because it was not published in the peer-reviewed literature.

[51] Ronald Simeone and Lynn Holland, *An Evaluation of Prescription Drug Monitoring Programs*, Simeone Associates, Inc., No. 2005PMBXK189, September 1, 2006, http://www.simeoneassociates.com/simeone3.pdf. This study was commissioned by the U.S. Department of Justice (DOJ), Office of Justice Programs (OJP), Bureau of Justice Assistance (BJA).

that while opioid abuse was increasing over time, the rate of increase was slower in states with PDMPs than in states without PDMPs.[52]

A 2014 briefing document from the Prescription Drug Monitoring Program Center of Excellence at Brandeis University (now called the PDMP Training and Technical Assistance Center) suggests that evidence shows PDMPs are "effective in improving clinical decision-making, reducing doctor shopping and diversion of controlled substances, and assisting in other efforts to curb the prescription drug abuse epidemic."[53] In 2015, the University of Kentucky Institute for Pharmaceutical Outcomes and Policy examined the effectiveness of mandatory enrollment of prescribers and dispensers in PDMPs in Kentucky and cited closures of non-physician-owned pain management facilities and a decrease (over 50%) in the number of individuals doctor shopping as two of several positive outcomes from mandatory reporting in Kentucky.[54]

Several more recently published articles reported positive results for prescription drug monitoring programs. In one article, researchers found that implementation of state PDMPs, in particular those with "robust characteristics,"[55] was associated with a modest reduction in opioid-related overdose deaths.[56] Another study found that states with prescription drug monitoring mandates were associated with a 9% to 10% reduction in population-adjusted numbers of Schedule II opioid prescriptions received by Medicaid enrollees and similar reductions in Medicaid spending on

---

[52] Liza M. Reifler et al., "Do Prescription Monitoring Programs Impact State Trends in Opioid Abuse/Misuse," *Pain Medicine*, no. 13 (2012), pp. 434-442.

[53] Prescription Drug Monitoring Program Center of Excellence at Brandeis (now called the PDMP Training and Technical Assistance Center), *Briefing on PDMP Effectiveness*, updated September 2014, p. 3.

[54] Patricia R. Freeman, Amie Goodin, and SuZanne Troske, et al., *Kentucky House Bill 1 Impact Evaluation*, Kentucky House Bill 1 Impact Evaluation, Prepared for The Kentucky Cabinet for Health and Family Services, March 2015.

[55] Robust characteristics include monitoring greater numbers of drugs with abuse potential and updating PDMP data at least weekly.

[56] Using an interrupted time-series analysis, the authors found that a state's implementation of a PDMP was associated with an average reduction of 1.12 opioid-related overdose deaths per 100,000 population in each state in the year after implementation. States whose programs had "robust characteristics" had greater reductions in deaths, compared to states whose programs did not have these characteristics. See Stephen W. Patrick, Carrie E. Fry, and Timothy F. Jones et al., "Implementation Of Prescription Drug Monitoring Programs Associated With Reductions In Opioid-Related Death Rates," *Health Affairs*, vol. 35, no. 7 (July 2016), pp. 1324-1332.

these prescriptions.[57] A third study reported no associations between PDMP implementation and nonmedical initiation/abuse of opioids, but did report a significant association between PDMP implementation and a reduction in "doctor shopping."[58]

Research shows that PDMPs may have positive effects beyond their intended purpose. For example, when accessing information from a PDMP, a prescriber or dispenser may identify a patient who is receiving legitimate prescriptions for multiple controlled substances and who is therefore at risk of harmful drug interactions.[59] PDMPs may also enable prescribers to monitor their own U.S. Drug Enforcement Administration (DEA) number to determine whether someone else is using it to forge prescriptions.[60]

Limitations of the Research

Research regarding PDMP effectiveness is limited, at least in part, by the difficulties inherent in conducting such research. Challenges in conducting high-quality research on PDMP effectiveness include (but are not limited to) (1) defining effectiveness, (2) accounting for differences among PDMPs, and (3) considering potential confounding factors.

To study effectiveness, researchers must first define effectiveness in a way that can be systematically measured as a study outcome. Almost all PDMPs are statewide programs; thus, researchers look for outcome measures for which statewide data are available. Some outcomes that have

---

[57] A reduction in opioid prescriptions may or may not be viewed as a positive effect. This association was observed largely with mandates of registration in PDMPs and not with mandates of use. See Wen Hefei, Bruce R. Schackman, and Brandom Aden et al., "States With Prescription Drug Monitoring Mandates Saw A Reduction In Opioids Prescribed To Medicaid Enrollees," *Health Affairs*, vol. 36, no. 4 (April 2017), pp. 733-741.

[58] Mir M. Ali, William N. Dowd, and Timothy Classen et al., "Prescription drug monitoring programs, nonmedical use of prescription drugs, and heroin use: Evidence from the National Survey of Drug Use and Health," *Addictive Behaviors*, vol. 69 (June 2017), pp. 65-77.

[59] Some states may see this as an intended purpose of creating a PDMP. Jeanmarie Perrone and Lewis S. Nelson, "Medication Reconciliation for Controlled Substances—An 'Ideal' Prescription-Drug Monitoring Program," *New England Journal of Medicine*, vol. 366, no. 25 (2012), p. 2341-2343.

[60] Ibid.

been measured in research on PDMP effectiveness are shipments and sales of controlled substances, benzodiazepine use in a Medicaid population, opioid consumption, substance abuse treatment admissions, drug overdose mortality, and multiple provider episodes (i.e., doctor shopping).[61] One drawback of using opioid consumption as an outcome measure is that it includes both nonmedical use of opioids and medically appropriate use of opioids to manage pain. A limitation of using a count of substance abuse treatment admissions is that it fails to capture substance abuse that goes untreated. Each of these measures presents only a portion of the picture of prescription drug diversion and abuse.

Studies that compared states with and without PDMPs and/or before and after implementation of a PDMP vary in the degree to which they account for differences among PDMPs. For example, despite evidence that proactive PDMPs are more effective than reactive PDMPs, most studies do not distinguish between proactive and reactive PDMPs.[62] Another difference that may influence PDMP effectiveness is which drugs are required to be reported to the PDMP, ranging from only those prescription drugs with the highest potential for abuse to all prescription controlled substances plus other drugs of concern. Research generally focuses on those controlled substances that are included in all of the PDMPs being examined. Differences in PDMPs over time may also influence effectiveness. For example, some states have transitioned from paper-based systems for monitoring prescriptions for controlled substances to the electronic PDMPs used today. Effectiveness studies have generally not accounted for such transitions over time, classifying two different systems as the same PDMP. Accounting for these and other differences between PDMPs may shed light on factors that influence effectiveness.

---

[61] See summaries of several studies conducted between 2001 and 2011 in Julie Worley, "Prescription Drug Monitoring Programs, a Response to Doctor Shopping: Purpose, Effectiveness, and Directions for Future Research," *Issues in Mental Health Nursing*, vol. 33, no. 5 (2012), pp. 319-328; see also Liza M. Reifler et al., "Do Prescription Monitoring Programs Impact State Trends in Opioid Abuse/Misuse," *Pain Medicine*, vol. 13, no. 3 (2012), pp. 434-442; and Aaron M. Gilson et al., "Time Series Analysis of California's Prescription Monitoring Program: Impact on Prescribing and Multiple Provider Episodes," *Journal of Pain*, vol. 13, no. 2 (2012), pp. 103-111.

[62] Proactive PDMPs send out unsolicited reports to authorized users, while reactive PDMPs send solicited reports.

Researchers also contend with factors that may confound study results, both when comparing outcomes across states and when comparing outcomes over time. For example, the baseline rate of prescription drug abuse may vary across states. The authors of a previously referenced study noted that the likelihood of abuse was actually higher in states with PDMPs than in states without PDMPs, but that proactive PDMPs inhibited the rate of increase in prescription drug abuse.[63] A PDMP may be part of a larger effort to reduce prescription drug diversion and abuse, in which case other initiatives may be responsible for any change in the outcome. A seemingly unrelated event, such as an economic downturn or upturn, may also affect the outcome. These considerations, among many others, impede the ability of researchers—and therefore policymakers—to draw conclusions about the effectiveness of PDMPs.

Potential Unintended Consequences

PDMPs may have unintended consequences beyond reducing prescription drug diversion and abuse.[64] Prescribers may hesitate to prescribe medications monitored by the PDMP—even for appropriate medical use—if they are concerned about potentially coming under scrutiny from law enforcement or licensing authorities.[65] Studies of paper-based prescription monitoring programs that preceded the electronic PDMPs found that many prescribers did not order the required prescription forms, rendering them unable to prescribe specified controlled substances. Their concerns may lead prescribers to replace medications that are

---

[63] Ronald Simeone and Lynn Holland, *An Evaluation of Prescription Drug Monitoring Programs*, Simeone Associates, Inc., No. 2005PMBXK189, September 1, 2006, http://www.simeoneassociates.com/simeone3.pdf.

[64] Most of the unintended consequences identified in this section are discussed in Scott M. Fishman et al., "Regulating Opioid Prescribing Through Prescription Monitoring Programs: Balancing Drug Diversion and Treatment of Pain," *Pain Medicine*, vol. 5, no. 3 (2004), pp. 309-324.

[65] Some have indicated that doctors hesitate to prescribe due to fear of scrutiny. See M. Mofizul Islam and Ian S. McRae, "An inevitable wave of prescription drug monitoring programs in the context of prescription opioids: pros, cons and tensions," *BMC Pharmacology & Toxicology*, vol. 15 (August 16, 2014); and Linda A. Johnson,"Americans Are Filling Fewer Prescriptions for Opioids Amid Rising Fear of Addiction," *TIME*, April 19, 2018.

monitored by the PDMP with medications that are not monitored by the PDMP, even if the unmonitored medications are inferior in terms of effectiveness or side effects.

Like prescribers, patients may fear coming under scrutiny from law enforcement if they use medications monitored by the PDMP, even if they have a legitimate medical need for the medications.[66] Patients may worry about changes in prescribing behavior, which may limit their access to needed medications. Patients may worry about the additional cost of more frequent office visits if prescribers become more cautious about writing prescriptions with refills. Patients may also have concerns about the privacy and security of their prescription information if it is submitted to a PDMP.

Another potential unintended consequence of a state PDMP is that it may push drug diversion activities over the border into a neighboring state.[67] A GAO study, completed in 2002, identified evidence of this spillover across state lines.[68] This concern is one of the reasons interstate data sharing and interoperability have become priorities. Similarly, a PDMP may push drug diversion activities into a neighboring state with a PDMP that does not monitor as many medications. In any of these cases, the effectiveness of the PDMP may be offset by unintended consequences.

An additional possible unintended consequence of state PDMP activity may be an uptick in the abuse of nonprescription opioids such as heroin and illicit fentanyl. As mentioned, some academic and government experts link the comparatively higher cost of prescription drugs and the crackdown on prescription drug abuse to the recent rise in heroin abuse.[69]

---

[66] M. Mofizul Islam and Ian S. McRae, "An inevitable wave of prescription drug monitoring programs in the context of prescription opioids: pros, cons and tensions," *BMC Pharmacology & Toxicology*, vol. 15 (August 16, 2014).

[67] Given that all states now have an operational PDMP within their borders, this may not be as much of a concern, but it is possible that a similar effect may be found with neighboring states that have varying mandates of use, etc.

[68] U.S. General Accounting Office, *Prescription Drugs: State Monitoring Programs Provide Useful Tool to Reduce Diversion*, GAO-02-634, May 2002, p. 3, http://www.gao.gov/assets/240/234687.pdf.

[69] Pradip K. Muhuri, Joseph C. Gfroerer, and M. Christine Davies, *Associations of Nonmedical Pain Reliever Use and Initiation of Heroin Use in the United States*, Substance Abuse and Mental Health Services Administration, Center for Behavioral Health Statistics and Quality, August 2013, http://www.samhsa.gov/data/2k13/DataReview/DR006/ nonmedical-pain-

A PDMP may also have positive unintended consequences. For example, when accessing information from a PDMP, a prescriber or dispenser may identify a patient who is receiving legitimate prescriptions for multiple controlled substances and who is therefore at risk of harmful drug interactions.[70] PDMPs may also enable prescribers to monitor their own U.S. Drug Enforcement Administration (DEA) number to determine whether someone else is using it to forge prescriptions.[71]

Potential to Increase Effectiveness

In 2012, the PDMP Center of Excellence at Brandeis University (now called the PDMP Training and Technical Assistance Center) published PDMP best practices and evaluated the quality of evidence supporting each best practice candidate.[72] Most of the best-practice candidates were supported by the weakest of five possible levels of evidence:[73]

1. randomized controlled trial or meta-analysis (0 best-practice candidates)
2. observational study with comparison groups (2 best-practice candidates)

---

reliever-use-2013.pdf; Theodore J. Cicero, Matthew S. Ellis, and Hilary L. Surratt, "Effect of Abuse- Deterrent Formulation of Oxycontin," *New England Journal of Medicine*, vol. 367, no. 2 (July 12, 2012), pp. 187-189;

U.S. Department of Justice, National Drug Intelligence Center, *National Drug Threat Assessment 2003*, "Narcotics", January 2003, http://www.justice.gov/archive/ndic/pubs3/3300/pharm.htm; and U.S. Department of Justice, National Drug Intelligence Center, *National Drug Threat Assessment 2011*, August 2011, p. 37, http://www.justice.gov/archive/ ndic/pubs44/44849/44849p.pdf.

[70] Some states may see this as an intended purpose of creating a PDMP. Jeanmarie Perrone and Lewis S. Nelson, "Medication Reconciliation for Controlled Substances—An "Ideal" Prescription-Drug Monitoring Program," *New England Journal of Medicine*, vol. 366, no. 25 (2012), p. 2341-2343.

[71] Ibid.

[72] Prescription Drug Monitoring Program Center of Excellence (now called the PDMP Training and Technical Assistance Center), *Prescription Drug Monitoring Programs: An Assessment of the Evidence for Best Practices*, September 20, 2012.

[73] In this list, best-practice candidates supported by more than one level of evidence are assigned to the strongest level of evidence.

3. observational study without comparison group (6 best-practice candidates)
4. case study or written documentation of expert opinion (6 best-practice candidates)
5. accumulated experience and/or key stakeholder perceptions (21 best-practice candidates)

A PDMP is essentially a source of information; its effectiveness depends largely on the quality of the information and how the information is used.[74] The quality of PDMP information depends on its timeliness, completeness, accuracy, and consistency. Expert recommendations to enhance data quality include

- collecting data at the point of sale (in real time);
- monitoring all prescribed controlled substances and other drugs of concern;
- integrating electronic prescribing technology;
- sharing data between states;
- standardizing the content across states;
- identifying the person picking up the prescription (which may be someone other than the patient, such as a family member); and
- linking prescription records for an individual (to avoid confusion if, for example, an address changes or a name is spelled differently).

For PDMP information to be well used, it must be accessible. A survey of prescribers found that the most common reason given for not using a PDMP was the time required to access it (73%); two other reasons—difficulty navigating the web portal (29%) and forgetting the password

[74] See Prescription Drug Monitoring Program Center of Excellence (now called the PDMP Training and Technical Assistance Center), *Prescription Drug Monitoring Programs: An Assessment of the Evidence for Best Practices*; and

(2) Jeanmarie Perrone and Lewis S. Nelson, "Medication Reconciliation for Controlled Substances—An "Ideal" Prescription-Drug Monitoring Program," *New England Journal of Medicine*, vol. 366, no. 25 (2012), p.2341-2343.

(28%)—may contribute to the amount of time required to access PDMP information. More than a third of survey respondents (39%) felt that accessing PDMP information would not change their prescribing practices for their patients, although research suggests PDMP information changes prescribing behavior. Relatively small numbers of respondents reported that lack of computer availability (9%) or never having applied for access (11%) were barriers to using a PDMP.[75] Expert recommendations to enhance data use include

- providing easy online access;
- issuing automated, unsolicited reports; and
- increasing participation through education and promotional campaigns.

Experts recommend making PDMP information available for research and public health purposes, which would require permitting access by designated nonprescribers (e.g., researchers and medical examiners). An example of a public health use of PDMP information is to identify patients for enrollment in special programs: Washington state used its PDMP to select Medicaid enrollees for a Patient Review Coordination Program, which decreased emergency department visits, physician visits, and prescriptions (resulting in an average savings of $6,000 per patient per year).[76] PDMP data may also be analyzed to identify geographic areas where interventions (such as increased law enforcement attention or establishment of a substance abuse clinic) are most needed. Carefully controlled access to de-identified data for research and public health purposes may yield other uses.

---

[75] Jeanmarie Perrone and Lewis S. Nelson, "Medication Reconciliation for Controlled Substances—An "Ideal" Prescription-Drug Monitoring Program," *New England Journal of Medicine*, vol. 366, no. 25 (2012), p. 2341-2343.

[76] Washington state update presented at Harold Rogers PDMP National Meeting, Washington, DC, June 4-6, 2012.

FEDERAL PROGRAMS THAT SUPPORT STATE PDMPS

The federal government supports state PDMPs through programs at the Departments of Justice (DOJ) and Health and Human Services (HHS). Since FY2002, DOJ has administered the Harold Rogers Prescription Drug Monitoring Program, and in FY2017, DOJ incorporated this grant program into the new Comprehensive Opioid Abuse Program. HHS programs include the National All Schedules Prescription Electronic Reporting (NASPER), State Demonstration Grants for Comprehensive Opioid Abuse Response, Opioid Prevention in States grants, and various pilots and initiatives under the Office of the National Coordinator for Health Information Technology (ONC).

Harold Rogers PDMP—Comprehensive Opioid Abuse Grant Program

From FY2002 to FY2016, the Harold Rogers PDMP was a discretionary, competitive grant program administered by the U.S. Department of Justice (DOJ), Office of Justice Programs (OJP), Bureau of Justice Assistance (BJA). It was created to help law enforcement,[77] regulatory entities, and public health officials analyze data on prescriptions for controlled substances. In FY2017, DOJ incorporated the Harold Rogers PDMP into the new Comprehensive Opioid Abuse Grant Program, which was created under Section 201 of the Comprehensive Addiction and Recovery Act (CARA; P.L. 114-198). Prescription drug monitoring activities were authorized as a purpose area of the program.[78]

---

[77] Law enforcement uses of PDMP data include (but are not limited to) investigations of physicians who prescribe controlled substances for drug dealers or abusers, pharmacists who falsify records in order to sell controlled substances, and people who forge prescriptions. See U.S. Department of Justice, Drug Enforcement Administration, Office of Diversion Control, http://www.deadiversion.usdoj.gov.

[78] Specifically, Section 201 of CARA states, "From amounts made available to carry out this part, the Attorney General may make grants to States, units of local government, and Indian tribes, for use by the State, unit of local government, or Indian tribe to provide services primarily relating to opioid abuse, including for any one or more of the following...

Grant Purpose Areas

The program assists states (including U.S. territories and federally recognized tribal governments) in the planning, implementation, and enhancement of their PDMPs. This involves

- facilitating the exchange of information among states using technical solutions compliant with PMIX architecture;
- developing a training program for system users;
- assessing the efficiency and effectiveness of existing PDMPs and related initiatives;
- enhancing collaboration between law enforcement, prosecutors, treatment professionals, medical community members, and pharmacies to create a comprehensive PDMP strategy; and
- other authorized activities under the Comprehensive Opioid Abuse Grant Program.[79]

The Comprehensive Opioid Abuse Grant Program also offers training and technical assistance grants to promote the use of PDMPs.[80]

Appropriations

The Harold Rogers PDMP began receiving federal funding in FY2002 through the Departments of Commerce, Justice, and State, the Judiciary, and Related Agencies Appropriations Act, 2002 (P.L. 107-77). While the

---

(6) In the case of a State, developing, implementing, or expanding a prescription drug monitoring program to collect and analyze data related to the prescribing of schedules II, III, and IV controlled substances through a centralized database administered by an authorized State agency, which includes tracking the dispensation of such substances, and providing for interoperability and data sharing with each other such program in each other State, and with any interstate entity that shares information between such programs." Prescription drug monitoring is one of 10 purpose areas for this program listed in statute.

[79] U.S. Department of Justice, Office of Justice Programs, Bureau of Justice Assistance, *Comprehensive Opioid Abuse Site-based Program FY2017 Competitive Grant Announcement*, pp.17-18, https://www.bja.gov/Funding/CARA17.pdf (hereinafter, *Comprehensive Opioid Abuse Site-based Program FY 2017 Competitive Grant Announcement*).

[80] See U.S. Department of Justice, Office of Justice Programs, Bureau of Justice Assistance, *Comprehensive Opioid Abuse Program Training and Technical Assistance (TTA) Program FY 2017 Competitive Grant Announcement*, https://www.bja.gov/Funding/COAPTTA17.pdf.

program itself has never been authorized in statute, funding for the program was provided to DOJ each year through the annual appropriations process. Annual appropriations information is listed in Table 1. In FY2017, DOJ incorporated the Harold Rogers PDMP into the new Comprehensive Opioid Abuse Grant Program, and $14 million was appropriated for prescription drug monitoring as part of the broader DOJ "Opioids Initiative." In FY2018, the Consolidated Appropriations Act, 2018 (P.L. 115-141) more than doubled the amount for prescription drug monitoring[81] and provided $30 million for this purpose.

National All Schedules Prescription Electronic Reporting Act of 2005 (NASPER)

The NASPER PDMP grant was a formula grant administered by HHS, Substance Abuse and Mental Health Services Administration (SAMHSA), Center for Substance Abuse Treatment (CSAT).[82] NASPER grants were last funded in FY2010. NASPER was first authorized by the National All Schedules Prescription Electronic Reporting Act of 2005 (P.L. 109-60, NASPER), which amended the Public Health Service Act to require the Secretary of HHS to award grants to states[83] to establish or improve PDMPs. It was amended and reauthorized under Section 109 of the Comprehensive Addiction and Recovery Act of 2016 (CARA, P.L. 114-198). Since FY2010, funds have not been specifically appropriated for this program.

---

[81] Appropriations statute specifies that funds can be used to monitor scheduled listed chemical products in addition to prescription drugs.

[82] Unless otherwise noted, all information in this section on NASPER comes from 42 U.S.C. §280g-3.

[83] For purposes of NASPER, the term "State" is defined at 42 U.S.C. §280g-3(m)(8) to mean as "each of the 50 States, the District of Columbia, and any commonwealth or territory of the United States."

Table 1. Harold Rogers PDMP—Comprehensive Opioid Abuse Grant Program Funding through FY2018 (In millions of dollars)

Fiscal Year	Appropriation
2002	$2.00
2003	$7.50
2004	$7.00
2005	$10.00
2006	$7.50
2007	$7.50
2008	$7.05
2009	$7.00
2010	$7.00
2011	$5.80
2012	$7.00
2013	$6.51
2014	$7.00
2015	$11.00
2016	$13.00
2017[a]	$14.00
2018[a]	$30.00

Source: FY2002 data from P.L. 107-77; FY2003 data from P.L. 108-7; FY2004 data from P.L. 108-199; FY2005 data from P.L. 108-447; FY2006 data from P.L. 109-108; FY2007 data from P.L. 110-5; FY2008 data from P.L. 110-161; FY2009 data from P.L. 111-8; FY2010 data from P.L. 111-117; FY2011 data are based on CRS analysis of the text of P.L. 112-10; FY2012 data from P.L. 112-55. FY2013 data were provided by the Department of Justice. FY2014-FY2018 data were taken from the joint explanatory statements to accompany P.L. 113-76, P.L. 113-235, P.L. 114-113, P.L. 115-31 and P.L. 115-141.

[a]In FY2017, DOJ incorporated the Harold Rogers PDMP into the new Comprehensive Opioid Abuse Grant Program. In FY2017, $14 million was appropriated to monitor prescription drugs and scheduled listed chemical products as part of the broader appropriation for "comprehensive opioid abuse reduction activities." In FY2018, $30 million was appropriated to monitor prescription drugs and scheduled listed chemical products ag"

Grant Purpose Areas

The two objectives of NASPER are to (1) foster the establishment of state-administered PDMPs that providers can access for the early identification of patients at risk for addiction in order to initiate appropriate interventions, and (2) establish a set of best practices for new PDMPs and improvement of existing PDMPs.

Appropriations

The NASPER Act of 2005 authorized appropriations for NASPER for FY2006-FY2010. The program was funded in FY2009 and FY2010. The final continuing resolution for FY2011 (P.L. 112-10) specifically prohibited the funding of NASPER.[84] Section 109 of CARA authorized appropriations for NASPER for FY2017-FY2021; however, no funds have been appropriated for the program. In FY2018, while no funds were *specifically* appropriated for NASPER, Congress directed the Centers for Disease Control and Prevention (CDC) to promote the use of PDMPs, including implementation of activities described in NASPER as part of its opioid prescription drug overdose (PDO) prevention activity.[85] Annual authorizations of appropriations and actual appropriations are listed in Table 2.

To be eligible for NASPER grant funding, states must meet certain requirements, such as having legal authority to implement PDMPs. All states that submit applications and meet the requirements receive grants noncompetitively. The amount awarded to each state is defined by a two-part formula:[86]

1. Each state receives a base amount of 1% of the total funding (i.e., $20,000 in FY2010).
2. The remaining amount is distributed according to the ratio of the number of pharmacies in the individual state to the number of pharmacies in all states with approved applications.

The HHS Secretary may adjust a state's allotment after taking into consideration the budget cost estimate for its PDMP. Thirteen states received grants under NASPER in FY2010, the last year of funding.[87]

---

[84] Department of Defense and Full-Year Continuing Appropriations Act, 2011 (P.L. 112-10 §1815(a)(2)).

[85] Explanatory text to accompany P.L. 115-141.

[86] 42 U.S.C. §280g-3(a)(2)

[87] U.S. Department of Health and Human Services, *TAGGS - Tracking Accountability in Government Grants System*, http://taggs.hhs.gov/AdvancedSearch.cfm.

Table 2. National All Schedules Prescription Electronic Reporting Act of 2005 (NASPER) Funding through FY2018 (In millions of dollars)

Fiscal Year	Authorization of Appropriation	Appropriation
2006	$15.00	$0.00
2007	$15.00	$0.00
2008	$10.00	$0.00
2009	$10.00	$2.00
2010	$10.00	$2.00
2011	NA	$0.00
2012	NA	$0.00
2013	NA	$0.00
2014	NA	$0.00
2015	NA	$0.00
2016	NA	$0.00
2017	$10.00	$0.00
2018	$10.00	$0.00[a]

Sources: Authorizations of appropriations for FY2006-FY2010 from P.L. 109-60, and authorizations of appropriations for FY2017 (through FY2021, not shown) are from P.L. 114-198. Appropriations for FY2006- FY2010 are from SAMHSA's Justification of Estimates for Appropriations Committees for FY2011. Appropriations for subsequent years are from P.L. 112-10, P.L. 112-74, P.L. 113-6. P.L. 113-76, P.L. 113-235, P.L. 114-113, P.L. 115-31, and P.L. 115-141.

Note: NA = not authorized.

[a]In FY2018, while no funds were directly appropriated for NASPER, Congress directed the Centers for Disease Control and Prevention to promote the use of PDMPs, including implementation of activities described in NASPER. This direction was provided under the heading "Opioid Prescription Drug Overdose (PDO) Prevention Activity," for which Congress appropriated $475.58 million. See Division H of the explanatory text to accompany the Consolidated Appropriations Act, 2018 (P.L. 115-141).

Although NASPER is not currently funded, HHS continues to support state PDMPs through other programs. For example, since 2015, the CDC has awarded funding to some states for PDO prevention activities, including efforts to improve access to PDMPs and the timeliness of PDMP data.[88]

---

[88] HHS, CDC, *Prescription Drug Overdose Prevention for States*, https://www.cdc.gov/drugoverdose/states/ state_prevention.html.

Program Comparison

Table 3 provides an overview and comparison of the Harold Rogers PDMP and the NASPER PDMP. Basic information is provided on program legislation, administering agencies, program objectives, grant types, authorization of appropriations, and actual appropriations.

Table 3. Comparison of the Harold Rogers PDMP - Comprehensive Opioid Abuse Grant Program and NASPER

	Harold Rogers[a]	**NASPER**
Legislation	Departments of Commerce, Justice, and State, the Judiciary, and Related Agencies Appropriations Act, 2002 (P.L. 107-77); and the Comprehensive Addiction and Recovery Act of 2016 (P.L. 114-198).	National All Schedules Prescription Electronic Reporting Act of 2005 (P.L. 109-60), amended by the Comprehensive Addiction and Recovery Act of 2016 (P.L. 114-198)
Administering Agency	U.S. Department of Justice (DOJ), Office of Justice Programs (OJP), Bureau of Justice Assistance (BJA)	U.S. Department of Health and Human Services (HHS), Substance Abuse and Mental Health Services Administration (SAMHSA), Center for Substance Abuse Treatment (CSAT)
Program Objectives	Help states to plan, implement, and enhance their PDMPs.	Two objectives: 1. Foster the establishment of state-administered PDMPs that providers can access for the early identification of patients at risk for addiction in order to initiate appropriate interventions. 2. Establish a set of best practices for new programs and improvement of existing programs.
Grant Types	Discretionary, competitive grants for states that have a pending or enacted enabling statute or regulation requiring the submission of controlled substance prescription data to an authorized state agency.	Formula grant program in which each state with an approved application receives funding according to the following two-part formula: 1. Each state receives a base amount of 1% of the total funding.

Table 3. (Continued)

	Harold Rogers[a]	NASPER
	Cities, counties, or regions within states that do not have an enabling state statute requiring the submission of PDMP data to an authorized state agency are eligible to apply under certain conditions.	2. The remaining amount is distributed according to the ratio of the number of pharmacies in the individual state to the number of pharmacies in all states with approved applications. The HHS Secretary may adjust the amount allocated to a state, after taking into consideration the estimated cost of the state's PDMP.
Authorization of Appropriations	From FY2002 to FY2016, the program itself was not authorized in statute while funding for the program was provided to DOJ each year since FY2002 through the annual appropriations process. In FY2017, DOJ incorporated the Harold Rogers PDMP into the new Comprehensive Opioid Abuse Grant Program, which was authorized at $103.00 million per year for FY2017-FY2021.	Authorizes to be appropriated $15.00 million per year for FY2006-FY2007, $10.00 million per year for FY2008-FY2010, and $10.00 million per year for FY2017-FY2021.
Appropriations	Appropriated $2.00 million in FY2002, $7.50 million in FY2003, $7.00 million in FY2004, $10.00 million in FY2005, $7.50 million in FY2006, $7.50 million in FY2007, $7.05 million in FY2008, $7.00 million in FY2009, $7.00 million in FY2010, $5.8 million in FY2011, $7.00 million in FY2012, $6.51 million in FY2013, $7.00 million in FY2014,	No funds were appropriated for FY2006- FY2008; appropriated $2.00 million per year in FY2009 and FY2010;

	Harold Rogers[a]	NASPER
	$11.00 million in FY2015, $13.00 million in FY2016, $14.00 million in FY2017, and $30.00 million in FY2018	funding prohibited in final continuing resolution for FY2011; no funds were appropriated for FY2012-FY2018.

Source: CRS summary of information from the following sources:

For the Harold Rogers PDMP, CRS summary of U.S. Department of Justice, Bureau of Justice Assistance, Comprehensive Opioid Abuse Grant Program, https://www.bja.gov. For appropriations, see source list for Table 1. For authorization, see Section 109 of the Comprehensive Addiction and Recovery Act of 2016 (P.L. 114-198).

For NASPER authorization, see CRS summary of the National All Schedules Prescription Electronic Reporting Act of 2005 (P.L. 109-60); Section 109 of the Comprehensive Addiction and Recovery Act of 2016 (P.L. 114- 198); and SAMHSA's Justification of Estimates for Appropriations Committees for FY2011. For appropriations, see source list for Table 2.

[a]While DOJ incorporated the Harold Rogers PDMP into the new Comprehensive Opioid Abuse Grant Program, it is still generally referred to as the Harold Rogers PDMP.

Other Programs

Other federal programs that are explicitly used to support PDMPs include Opioid Prevention in States, PDMPs and Health Information Technology (IT), State Demonstration Grants for Comprehensive Opioid Abuse Response, and State Targeted Response to the Opioid Crisis Grants—all of which are administered by HHS.

Opioid Prevention in States

Opioid Prevention in States (OPIS) is the umbrella term for all opioid grants administered by CDC. The OPIS grants fall under CDC's Center for Injury Prevention and Control. Among the OPIS grant programs, two require states to use funds for PDMPs: the Prevention for States (PfS) grants and the Data-Driven Prevention Initiative (DDPI). Since 2015, CDC has awarded PfS funding to some states for prescription drug overdose prevention activities, including efforts to improve access to PDMPs and the timeliness of PDMP data.[89] Since 2016, CDC has awarded DDPI funding to some states and the District of Columbia to help them with

89 HHS, CDC, *Prevention for States*, https://www.cdc.gov/drugoverdose/states/state_prevention.html.

opioid-related data collection and analysis; strategies to change behaviors driving prescription opioid abuse; and overdose prevention programs.[90]

These individual grant programs are not explicitly authorized in statute. The CDC Center for Injury Control and Prevention conducts activities authorized under numerous provisions, including general public health authorities of the HHS Secretary. The most directly relevant is Public Health Service Act (PHSA) Section 392, which broadly authorizes CDC to provide assistance to states and localities for injury prevention and control, but does not include an explicit authorization of appropriations. According to CDC's FY2019 budget request, the PfS and DDPI grant awards together were funded at $72 million in both FY2017 and FY2018.[91]

PDMPs and Health IT

The Office of the National Coordinator for Health Information Technology (ONC) has undertaken efforts to support the integration of PDMPs with health IT and to enhance clinician access to PDMP information using health IT. These efforts included a series of pilots, in collaboration with SAMHSA, from 2011 to 2013 to test different approaches to increasing provider access to PDMP information through health IT. In addition, ONC has undertaken an initiative to develop approaches to the challenge of a lack of uniform standards for sharing PDMP data with health IT systems such as electronic health records (EHRs) and health information exchanges.

Although ONC has directed funding to support these efforts beginning as early as 2011, they are not specifically authorized in statute and instead appear to be carried out under general statutory authorities for ONC in Title XXX of the PHSA. Both the FY2016 and the FY2017 ONC Congressional Budget Justifications requested $5 million in each of those years for efforts to support PDMP and Health IT integration under the

---

90 HHS, CDC, *Data-Driven Prevention Initiative (DDPI)*, https://www.cdc.gov/drugoverdose/foa/ddpi.html.

91 HHS, CDC, *Justification of Estimates for Appropriation Committees* for FY2019, p. 221. The FY2018 amount presented was based on the annualized FY2017 continuing resolution. These were not line items in the CDC FY2017 operating plan.

broader budget category of Policy Development and Coordination.[92] These funds were to be used for activities including technical assistance for state PDMPs with HIT integration; challenge awards to design and use HIT to access PDMPs in clinical settings; and further adoption of electronic prescribing of controlled substances. The FY2018 and FY2019 ONC Congressional Budget Justifications do not specifically mention anything about efforts related to PDMPs.

State Demonstration Grants for Comprehensive Opioid Abuse Response

The State Demonstration Grants for Comprehensive Opioid Abuse Response were newly authorized for FY2017 by the Comprehensive Addiction and Recovery Act of 2016 (CARA, P.L. 114-198). CARA amended the PHSA by adding a new Section 548 requiring the HHS Secretary to "award grants to States, and combinations of States, to implement an integrated opioid abuse response initiative."[93] A state's response initiative may include "establishing, maintaining, or improving" a PDMP, as well as other elements such as efforts to provide education, and prevent and treat opioid abuse. PHSA Section 548 specifies that the HHS Secretary, in awarding these grants, shall give priority to a state meeting certain conditions, including several related to PDMPs (e.g., a state that ensures the capability of sharing PDMP data with other states).

PHSA Section 548 authorizes to be appropriated $5 million for the state demonstration grants for each of FY2017-FY2021. The state demonstration grants were not funded in FY2017 and FY2018.[94]

---

[92] HHS, ONC, *Justification of Estimates for Appropriations Committee* for FY2017, https://www.healthit.gov/sites/ default/files/final_onc_cj_fy_2017_clean.pdf, p. 30; and HHS, ONC, *Justification of Estimates for Appropriations Committee* for FY2016, https://www.healthit.gov/sites/default/files/ONC-FY2016-budget-justification.pdf, pp. 26-27.

[93] P.L. 114-198, §601.

[94] P.L. 115-31 and P.L. 115-141.

State Targeted Response to the Opioid Crisis Grants

SAMHSA's State Targeted Response to the Opioid Crisis Grants were newly authorized by the 21st Century Cures Act (Division A of P.L. 114-255; see Section 1003). One of several authorized purpose areas is improving state prescription drug monitoring programs. In FY2018, $1 billion was provided to SAMHSA for this grant program.[95]

The VA and PDMP Participation

Federal agencies that provide health care have faced some challenges in working with state PDMPs. For example, before the Department of Veterans Affairs (VA) could contribute prescription data to state PDMPs, a statutory change was necessary to authorize the VA Secretary to disclose relevant information; this change occurred in the Consolidated Appropriations Act, 2012 (P.L. 112-74, Title II, Section 230). Since then, the VA has worked state by state to be able to contribute data to each state's PDMP.

The VA has also worked state by state to enable VA prescribers to query each state's PDMP because, for example, some state PDMP laws may restrict registration to prescribers who are licensed in the state, and some VA prescribers are licensed in a state other than where they work for the VA. In October 2016, the VA issued a policy establishing minimum requirements for VA providers to query state PDMPs under specified circumstances such as prior to initiating therapy with a controlled substance (VHA Directive 1306).

SELECTED POLICY ISSUES

Role of PDMPs in Federal Efforts to Address Prescription Drug Abuse

In 2011, in response to the "epidemic"[96] of prescription drug abuse, the Obama Administration released an action plan.[97] This plan, from the Office

[95] See "Division H-Departments of Labor, Health and Human Services, and Education, and Related Agencies Appropriations Act, 2018," *Congressional Record*, vol. 164 (March 22, 2018), p. H2702.

[96] According to the National Survey on Drug Use and Health (NSDUH) in 2010, estimates of persons aged 12 and over who currently used "prescription-type psychotherapeutic drugs" nonmedically (7 million or 2.7% of this population) were similar to estimates in 2009 (7 million, or 2.8% of this population) and in 2002 (6.3 million, or 2.7% of this population). See SAMHSA, *Results from the 2010 National Survey on Drug Use and Health: Summary*

of National Drug Control Policy (ONDCP), outlined four primary areas that may reduce the abuse of prescription drugs: educating individuals on the safe use of prescription drugs and risks involved in abusing them; implementing prescription drug monitoring programs (PDMPs) in the states and encouraging information sharing; developing programs for proper drug disposal; and providing law enforcement with tools to enforce proper prescribing practices and disband "pill mills."[98]

As part of this plan, the Administration outlined actions to improve the functioning of state PDMPs and increase interstate PDMP operability and communications. Specific actions offered included

- working with states to establish effective PDMPs by encouraging research on PDMP effectiveness and means to improve PDMP effectiveness;
- supporting the NASPER reauthorization;
- ensuring that the Department of Veterans Affairs (VA)[99] and the Department of Defense (DOD)[100] are authorized to share patient information with state PDMPs;

---

of National Findings, p. 1. The Obama Administration pointed to statistics such as initiation of drug use, how people accessed prescription pain relievers, youth use of prescription drugs (at the time it was the second most-abused category of drugs after marijuana), and rising prescription drug abuse among active duty servicemembers.

97 Office of National Drug Control Policy, *Epidemic: Responding to America's Prescription Drug Abuse Crisis*, 2011.

98 "Pill mill" is a term used to describe a doctor, clinic, or pharmacy that is prescribing or dispensing narcotics inappropriately or for nonmedical reasons. They may be disguised as independent pain-management centers. They tend to open and shut down quickly to evade law enforcement.

99 The Consolidated Appropriations Act, 2012 (P.L. 112-74) authorized the VA Secretary to share prescription information with state PDMPs.

100 According to Department of Defense, *Report to Congress: Medication Management for Physically and Psychologically Wounded Armed Forces Members In Fiscal Year 2011-2012*, RefID: 6-B74CA6F, March 14, 2012, "DoD providers can access PDMPs for controlled substance prescription histories before generating prescriptions for controlled substances.... The military specific response to this challenge includes work by the PharmacoVigilance Center to apply the lessons learned and apply it to the military where relevant." The report does not indicate whether DOD dispensers contribute information to state PDMPs; however, if servicemembers fill prescriptions at retail pharmacies in the private sector (in a state with a PDMP), the prescriptions would be reported just like any others.

- encouraging federally funded health care programs to provide controlled substance prescription information to the state PDMPs (in states where they operate health care facilities or pharmacies);
- exploring the feasibility of reimbursing prescribers for checking PDMPs before writing controlled substance prescriptions to patients covered under insurance plans;
- evaluating programs that require certain doctor shoppers or drug abusing individuals to use one doctor and one pharmacy;
- evaluating the potential for state PDMPs to reduce Medicare and Medicaid fraud;
- issuing a final rule from DEA on electronic prescribing of controlled substances;
- increasing the use of "Screening, Brief Intervention, and Referral to Treatment" programs to identify and prevent prescription drug abuse;
- identifying how health information technologies can enhance prescription drug information;
- testing the usefulness of the Centers for Disease Control and Prevention's surveillance system to generate measures of prescription drug abuse;
- assessing the use of the Drug Abuse Warning Network to better understand prescription drug abuse at the community level;
- expanding DOJ's efforts to enhance interstate PDMP interoperability, particularly though the PMIX program; and
- evaluating existing databases with information on prescription drug access, use, misuse, and toxicity to improve their utility and as new sources of data.[101]

While this plan was never updated, the Obama Administration released a fact sheet in October 2015 outlining its public and private sector efforts

[101] The White House, *Epidemic: Responding to America's Prescription Drug Abuse Crisis*, 2011, pp. 6-7.

to address both prescription drug abuse and heroin use.[102] This fact sheet noted that President Obama had issued a memorandum to federal departments and agencies directing two essential elements in combating this problem: prescriber training and improving access to treatment. It went on to describe private sector efforts, which included the National Association of Boards of Pharmacy enhancing access to PDMP data to thousands more physicians and pharmacists in Arizona, Delaware, Kentucky, and North Dakota in 2016. It also went on to describe public sector efforts, which included the federal government expanding access to PDMP data throughout federal agencies.[103]

In 2017, President Trump established the President's Commission on Combating Drug Addiction and the Opioid Crisis, which has issued a report outlining recommendations to combat the opioid crisis. Among its recommendations, the commission issued two that were specific to PDMPs:

1. The Commission recommends the Administration's support of the Prescription Drug Monitoring (PDMP) Act to mandate states that receive grant funds to comply with PDMP requirements, including data sharing. This Act directs DOJ to fund the establishment and maintenance of a data-sharing hub.
2. The Commission recommends federal agencies mandate PDMP checks, and consider amending requirements under the Emergency Medical Treatment and Labor Act (EMTALA), which requires hospitals to screen and stabilize patients in an emergency department, regardless of insurance status or ability to pay.[104]

---

[102] The White House, *FACT SHEET: Obama Administration Announces Public and Private Sector Efforts to Address Prescription Drug Abuse and Heroin Use*, https://obamawhitehouse.archives.gov/the-press-office/2015/10/21/fact- sheet-obama-administration-announces-public-and-private-sector.

[103] Ibid.

[104] The President's Commission on Combating Drug Addiction and the Opioid Crisis, *Final Report*, November 1, 2017, pp. 53-54, https://www.whitehouse.gov/sites/whitehouse.gov/files/images/Final_Report_Draft_11-1-2017.pdf.

In regard to Recommendation #12, the Prescription Drug Monitoring Act of 2017 (H.R. 1854; S. 778) would, if enacted, require states receiving PDMP grant funds from DOJ or HHS[105] to comply with specified requirements, including a requirement to share their PDMP data with other states. Under the proposed legislation, DOJ and HHS may withhold grant funds from states that fail to comply. It also would direct DOJ to award a grant under the new Comprehensive Opioid Abuse Grant Program to establish and maintain an interstate data-sharing hub.

Supporting PDMPs is just one component in the overall federal effort against prescription drug abuse. Research on PDMP effectiveness has yielded sometimes inconclusive results on a number of desired outcomes, though research findings suggest that PDMPs may contribute to reduced doctor shopping and prescription drug abuse. As such, policymakers may want to assess the extent to which federal agencies' PDMP-related efforts have accomplished the Administration's goals to reduce illicit prescribing activities and prescription drug abuse.

Balancing Stakeholder Concerns

While establishment and enhancement of PDMPs (such as interstate data sharing and real-time data access) enjoy broad support,[106] some stakeholders express concerns about health care versus law enforcement uses of PDMP data, particularly with regard to protection of personally identifiable health information.

---

[105] Specifically, the bill references the Harold Rogers Prescription Drug Monitoring Program established under the Departments of Commerce, Justice, and State, the Judiciary, and Related Agencies Appropriations Act, 2002 and the controlled substance monitoring program under Section 399O of the Public Health Service Act.

[106] For example, the Pharmaceutical Research and Manufacturers of America (PhRMA)—the industry group representing pharmaceutical research and biotechnology companies—supports PDMPs and recommends assessing their effectiveness and exploring enhancements. PhRMA, *Prescription Drug Abuse*, http://www.phrma.org/prescription-drug-abuse.

Law Enforcement Use of PDMP Data[107]

Research has demonstrated that PDMPs save law enforcement officials time in investigations, *if law enforcement officials have access to PDMP information*. Concerns about potential law enforcement uses of PDMP data have been expressed by stakeholder organizations representing prescribers. The American Medical Association (AMA), a professional association of more than 200,000 physicians, supports the use of PDMPs and recommended that PDMPs be housed in health-related agencies (rather than law enforcement agencies).[108] AMA further recommends that information from PDMPs "be used first for education of the specific physicians involved prior to any civil action against these physicians."[109] The American Society of Addiction Medicine (ASAM), one of several national medical specialty societies under the AMA umbrella, likewise expresses concern about the use of PDMP data for purposes other than health care: "[L]aw enforcement, the judiciary, corrections professionals, employers, and others outside of the health care system should not be granted access to PDMP data except via the means available to them to secure access to other personally identifiable health information."[110] The fact that PDMPs contain personally identifiable health information raises concerns about privacy and data security. Both AMA and ASAM stress the need to subject PDMP information to the same standards applied to other patient records.[111]

---

[107] CRS Legislative Attorney Brian Yeh contributed to the legal discussion in this section.

[108] American Medical Association, *H-95.946 Prescription Drug Monitoring Program Confidentiality*, AMA Policy Statements, https://policysearch.ama-assn.org/policyfinder/detail/prescription%20drug%20monitoring%20program?uri=%2FAMADoc%2FHOD.xml-0-5325.xml.

[109] American Medical Association, *H-95.947 Prescription Drug Monitoring to Prevent Abuse of Controlled Substances*, AMA Policy Statements, https://policysearch.ama-assn.org/policyfinder/detail/prescription%20drug%20monitoring%20program?uri=%2FAMADoc%2FHOD.xml-0-5325.xml.

[110] American Society of Addiction Medicine (ASAM), *Public Policy Statement on Measures to Counteract Prescription Drug Diversion, Misuse and Addiction*, January 25, 2012, http://www.asam.org/advocacy/find-a-policy- statement/view-policy-statement/public-policy-statements/2012/01/26/measures-to-counteract-prescription-drug- diversion-misuse-and-addiction.

[111] American Medical Association, *H-95.946 Prescription Drug Monitoring Program Confidentiality*, AMA Policy Statements, https://policysearch.ama-assn.org/policyfinder/detail/prescription%20drug%20monitoring%20program? uri=%2FAMADoc%2FHOD.xml-

In recent years, to investigate violations of the federal Controlled Substances Act (CSA), the DEA has demanded access to certain PDMP data without a court order or search warrant, a practice that has caused some controversy[112] and been subject to court challenge.[113] The CSA contains a provision, 21 U.S.C. §876, that authorizes the DEA to issue administrative subpoenas (without prior court approval) to obtain documents that the agency finds are "relevant or material" to an investigation involving controlled substances.[114] The DEA may also seek judicial enforcement of such subpoenas "to compel compliance" with the requests for evidence.[115] In 2012, the Oregon Department of Justice filed a lawsuit against the DEA[116] in federal court seeking a declaratory judgment that, pursuant to state law,[117] the DEA must obtain "a valid court order" in order to access patient and physician records contained in the Oregon PDMP.[118] The DEA argued that the CSA's administrative subpoena provision preempts Oregon's statutory requirement.[119] Agreeing with the DEA, the U.S. Court of Appeals for the Ninth Circuit held that the CSA[120] preempted[121] the Oregon law because the provisions are in "positive conflict ... so that the two cannot consistently stand together."[122]

In another federal case, a Utah district court upheld the DEA's exercise of its administrative subpoena power to access the state's PDMP

0-5325.xml; and ASAM, *Public Policy Statement on Measures to Counteract Prescription Drug Diversion, Misuse and Addiction*, January 25, 2012, http://www.asam.org/advocacy/find-a-policy-statement/view-policy-statement/public-policy-statements/2012/01/26/measures-to-counteract-prescription-drug- diversion-misuse-and-addiction.

[112] Christian Gaston, "Oregon Sues DEA Over Access to Patient Drug Records," *The Oregonian*, November 30, 2012, http://www.oregonlive.com/politics/index.ssf/2012/11/oregon_sues_dea_over_access_to.html.

[113] This paragraph and the following one were authored by CRS Legislative Attorney Brian Yeh.

[114] 21 U.S.C. §876.

[115] 21 U.S.C. §876(c).

[116] Or. Prescription Drug Monitoring Program v. DEA, 998 F. Supp. 2d 957 (D. Or. 2014).

[117] Or. Rev. Stat. §431A.865(2)(a)(G) (2017).

[118] Or. Prescription Drug Monitoring Program v. DEA, 860 F.3d 1228, 1230 (9th Cir. 2017).

[119] Pursuant to the Supremacy Clause of Article VI of the U.S. Constitution, Congress has the power to preempt, or override, state law. U.S. Const. art. VI, cl. 2. The Controlled Substances Act contains a preemption provision codified at 21 U.S.C. §903.

[120] 21 U.S.C. §876.

[121] *Or. Prescription Drug Monitoring Program,* 860 F.3d at 1236.

[122] Ibid., quoting 21 U.S.C. §903.

database,[123] despite a Utah state law requirement that law enforcement officers may obtain such information only "pursuant to a valid search warrant."[124] Though the court first observed that the Supremacy Clause resolves the conflict between the conflicting federal and state laws at issue,[125] Utah asserted that the DEA's use of the CSA's administrative subpoena provision is not a "valid exercise of national power" because the Fourth Amendment's protections against unreasonable search and seizure require a search warrant to access the PDMP data.[126] The court disagreed with the state,[127] ruling that the DEA's subpoena authority is a valid exercise of national power "that does not offend the Fourth Amendment" because the pharmaceutical industry is a highly regulated one in which "physicians and patients have no reasonable expectation of privacy from the DEA" in the records stored in Utah's PDMP.[128]

Privacy of Individually Identifiable Health Information and PDMPs

PDMPs have elicited numerous concerns about patient privacy, including issues around the scope and breadth of authorized access to collected health information as well as the potential for unauthorized access or breaches. While PDMPs are seen as a valuable source of information in the effort to address improper prescribing of controlled substances, concerns exist about the potential deterrent effect on timely access to needed medication due to fears that sensitive health information

---

[123] United States Dep't of Justice v. Utah Dep't of Commerce, No. 2:16-cv-611-DN-DBP, 2017 U.S. Dist. LEXIS 118470 (D. Utah 2017).

[124] Utah Code Ann. §58-37f-301(2)(m) (LexisNexis 2017).

[125] *United States Dep't of Justice,* 2017 U.S. Dist. LEXIS 118470, at *16.

[126] Ibid. at *17.

[127] The Utah Attorney General's Office reportedly decided not to appeal the district court's decision. See Lindsay Whitehurst, "Utah to Obey Order for DEA Drug Database Search," *The Salt Lake Tribune*, August 22, 2017, https://www.sltrib.com/news/2017/08/22/utah-to-obey-order-for-dea-drug-database-search/.

[128] *United States Dep't of Justice,* 2017 U.S. Dist. LEXIS 118470, at *22. However, the court noted that Utah still has the authority to require a search warrant for *state and local* law enforcement officers and prosecutors to access the PDMP. Ibid. at *22.

will be shared with PDMPs, and may be subsequently legally disclosed or accessed through a breach.[129]

PDMPs have varying requirements with respect to the security and authorized use and disclosure of their stored information. These uses and disclosures are regulated by state law. PDMPs also receive protected health information (PHI) from pharmacists and other health care providers (HIPAA covered entities) who are subject to the federal HIPAA Privacy Rule.[130] In addition, individually identifiable health information that is generated pursuant to treatment at substance abuse facilities is subject to stricter privacy requirements established by the "Part 2" rule.[131]

The HIPAA Privacy Rule governs covered entities' (health care plans, providers and clearinghouses) and their business associates' use and disclosure of PHI. The rule describes multiple situations in which covered entities may use or disclose PHI, while all uses and disclosures of PHI by covered entities or business associates that are not expressly permitted under the rule require the individual's prior written authorization. Generally, covered entities may share PHI between and among themselves for the purposes of treatment, payment or healthcare operations, with few restrictions (and specifically, without out the individual's authorization).[132]

Certain other uses and disclosures (e.g., sharing PHI with family members and friends) are permitted, but require the covered entity to give the individual the opportunity to object or agree to the PHI's use or disclosure.[133]

The HIPAA Privacy Rule also recognizes that PHI may be useful in other circumstances aside from health care treatment and payment for a given individual. For this reason, the rule lists a number of "national priority purposes" for which covered entities may disclose PHI without an

---

[129] MM Islam, IS McRae, "An inevitable wave of prescription drug monitoring programs in the context of prescription opioids: pros, cons and tensions," BMC Pharmacological Toxicology, vol. 15, 2014.

[130] Protected health information is defined as individually identifiable health information that is transmitted by electronic media; maintained in electronic media; or transmitted or maintained in any other form or medium (45 C.F.R.§106.103).

[131] PHSA Section 543 (42 U.S.C. §290dd-2); 45 C.F.R. Part 2.

[132] 45 CFR §164.506

[133] 45 CFR §164.508, 45 CFR §164.510

individual's authorization or opportunity to agree or object.[134] PDMPs can receive PHI from covered entities under authority of one or more of these exceptions. Relevant exceptions include disclosures required by law—in this case, state PDMP laws; disclosures for public health activities; or disclosures for health oversight activities.

A PDMP is not a HIPAA covered entity, nor is it generally a business associate as defined by HIPAA, and in these cases the HIPAA requirements and standards for maintaining the security and privacy of the PHI—or for its re-disclosure—that apply to HIPAA covered entities would not apply to PDMPs. Although HIPAA may not apply, privacy and security requirements for PDMPs are still enumerated under state law.

Stricter privacy requirements—commonly known as the "Part 2" rule—apply at the federal level to individually identifiable patient information received or acquired by federally assisted substance abuse programs.[135] The "Part 2" rule allows such programs to disclose information with patient consent or pursuant to exceptions in regulation; however, in the case of PDMPs, it prohibits re-disclosure of information without patient consent. The requirement for consent may be a logistical deterrent to the submission of this information to PDMPs. In addition, since PDMPs are designed to share information with registered users, the "Part 2" rule's prohibition on re-disclosure without patient consent discourages federally assisted substance abuse programs from contributing to PDMPs' information about controlled substances dispensed for the treatment of opioid addiction (i.e., methadone or buprenorphine) due to concerns that authorized re- disclosures of the data could not be prevented.

Federal Role in Interstate Information Sharing and Interoperability

Federal policymakers have repeatedly emphasized the importance of enhancing interstate information sharing and the interoperability of state

[134] 45 CFR §164.512

[135] Stricter state privacy law may also apply on a state by state basis.

systems. The PDMP component of the Obama Administration's 2011 action plan to counter prescription drug abuse included efforts to improve the functioning of state PDMPs and increase interstate PDMP operability and communications. In 2013, HHS published a congressionally mandated report on PDMP interoperability standards for interstate exchange of PDMP information.[136] In November 2017, a presidential commission recommended, among other things, that the Trump Administration support legislation to require DOJ to fund a "data-sharing hub" and require states receiving federal grant funds to share PDMP data.[137]

The Rise in Illicit Opioid Abuse

In 2014, then-Attorney General Holder called the rise in heroin abuse "a sad but not unpredictable symptom of the significant increase in prescription drug abuse we've seen over the past decade."[138] While then-Attorney General Holder did not cite increased monitoring of prescription opioids and enforcement activities as a reason for the rise in heroin abuse, others have stated that the crackdown on prescription drug abuse may have led users to turn to heroin, a cheaper alternative to prescription drugs that may be more easily accessible to some who are seeking an opioid high.[139]

---

[136] HHS, *Prescription Drug Monitoring Program Interoperability Standards*, September 2013, https://www.healthit.gov/sites/default/files/fdasia1141report_final.pdf. The report was mandated by Section 1141(c) of P.L. 112-144

[137] The President's Commission on Combating Drug Addiction and the Opioid Crisis, *Final Report Draft*, November 1, 2017, p. 13, https://www.whitehouse.gov/sites/whitehouse.gov/files/images/Final_Report_Draft_11-1-2017.pdf.

[138] U.S. Department of Justice, *Attorney General Holder, Calling Rise in Heroin Overdoses 'Urgent Public Health Crisis,' Vows Mix of Enforcement, Treatment*, Justice News, March 10, 2014, http://www.justice.gov/opa/pr/2014/ March/14-ag-246.html.

[139] Pradip K. Muhuri, Joseph C. Gfroerer, and M. Christine Davies, *Associations of Nonmedical Pain Reliever Use and Initiation of Heroin Use in the United States*, Substance Abuse and Mental Health Services Administration, Center for Behavioral Health Statistics and Quality, August 2013, http://www.samhsa.gov/data/2k13/DataReview/DR006/ nonmedical-pain-reliever-use-2013.pdf; Theodore J. Cicero, Matthew S. Ellis, and Hilary L. Surratt, "Effect of Abuse- Deterrent Formulation of Oxycontin," *New England Journal of Medicine*, vol. 367, no. 2 (July 12, 2012), pp. 187-189;

U.S. Department of Justice, National Drug Intelligence Center, *National Drug Threat Assessment 2003*, "Narcotics", January 2003, http://www.justice.gov/archive/ndic/pubs3/3300/pharm.htm; and U.S. Department of Justice, National Drug Intelligence Center,

Policymakers may debate whether increased scrutiny and monitoring of prescription drug activity has unintentionally contributed to the increase in heroin abuse; and if this is the case, how might the government address this issue, if at all.

National Drug Threat Assessment 2011, August 2011, p. 37, http://www.justice.gov/archive/ ndic/pubs44/44849/44849p.pdf.

In: Prescription Drugs
Editor: Karen Sue McKinney
ISBN: 978-1-53617-288-1

Chapter 3

PRESCRIPTION OPIOIDS: PATIENT OPTIONS FOR SAFE AND EFFECTIVE DISPOSAL OF UNUSED OPIOIDS*

United States Government Accountability Office

ABBREVIATIONS

AMA	American Medical Association
CDC	Centers for Disease Control and Prevention
DEA	Drug Enforcement Administration
EPA	Environmental Protection Agency
FDA	Food and Drug Administration
REMS	risk evaluation and mitigation strategy
RCRA	Resource Conservation and Recovery Act
SAMHSA	Substance Abuse and Mental Health Services Administration
SUPPORT Act	SUPPORT for Patients and Communities Act

* This is an edited, reformatted and augmented version of United States Government Accountability Office, Report to Congressional Committees, Accessible Version, Publication No. GAO-19-650, dated September 2019.

Why GAO Did This Study

In 2017, an estimated 11.1 million Americans misused a prescription pain reliever, which included opioids. This misuse contributes to opioid abuse and death, which has quintupled from 1999 to 2017; about 17,000 people died from prescription opioid overdoses in 2017. Government agencies and stakeholders have attempted to address the potential for misuse and abuse by facilitating safe disposal of unused prescription opioids and other drugs.

The SUPPORT for Patients and Communities Act enacted in 2018 included a provision for GAO to review patient disposal of unused opioids, among other things. This chapter examines (1) federally recommended and other available methods patients may use to dispose of unused prescription opioids, and (2) what is known about patients' use of these methods.

To do this work, GAO examined peer-reviewed, academic literature on outcomes for prescription opioid disposal; reviewed federal agency documentation; interviewed federal agency officials, independent researchers, and stakeholder group representatives—such as those from the American Medical Association; and analyzed DEA data as of April 2019 on permanent drug collection sites. GAO also interviewed representatives of three companies that manufacture commercial in-home disposal products and reviewed publicly available documents about these products.

What GAO Found

The Food and Drug Administration (FDA), Drug Enforcement Administration (DEA), and Environmental Protection Agency (EPA) recommend that patients dispose of unused presciption opioids by bringing them to DEA-registered collection sites or a DEA take-back event, or using mail-back programs. As of April 2019, 70 percent of the U.S. population lived less than 5 miles from permanent collection sites, which are often located at pharmacies. If collection sites, take-back events, or mail-back programs are not feasible, FDA recommends quickly and permanently removing the most dangerous prescription opioids, such as hydrocodone and fentanyl, from the home by flushing them down the toilet. For all other prescription opioids, the agencies recommend disposal in the trash after mixing them with unpalatable substances, such as cat litter. Commercial products to facilitate in-home disposal also exist, and FDA is aware that patients may opt to use these products for disposal in the trash.

Available studies suggest that many patients are unaware of federally recommended disposal methods or choose not to dispose of unused prescription opioids. For example, five studies found that between one-quarter and three-quarters of patients stored unused opioids for future use or had misplaced their unused opioids. Further, federal data indicate that 85 percent of intentional misuse occurs with the patient's knowledge—for example, when a patient sells or gives away unused prescription opioids. To educate and motivate patients to dispose of unused opioids, FDA launched a public awareness campaign called "Remove the Risk" in April 2019. Also, FDA and other stakeholders have created educational materials for patients and providers on safe opioid disposal.

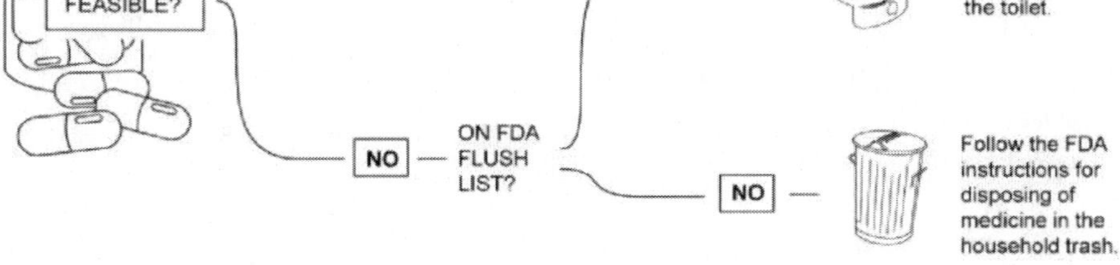

Source: GAO analysis of Food and Drug Administration (FDA) documents. | GAO-19-650.

FDA Recommendations for Disposal of Unused Prescription Opioids.

September 3, 2019

The Honorable Lamar Alexander
Chairman

The Honorable Patty Murray
Ranking Member
Committee on Health, Education, Labor, and Pensions
United States Senate

The Honorable Frank Pallone Jr.
Chairman

The Honorable Greg Walden
Republican Leader
Committee on Energy and Commerce
House of Representatives

The Substance Abuse and Mental Health Services Administration (SAMHSA) estimates that in 2017, 11.1 million people aged 12 or older used a prescription pain reliever, which includes opioids, in a way not intended by the prescriber.[1] Health care providers prescribe opioids to treat chronic pain and after an acute medical event, such as a surgery, to help patients manage pain while they heal.[2] Because patients may not take all of the opioids that their providers prescribe, many possess excess opioids that could be misused by the patient or someone else. This misuse contributes

---

[1] SAMHSA. *Key Substance Use and Mental Health Indicators in the United States: Results from the 2017 National Survey on Drug Use and Health*, (2018). Misuse of prescription opioids includes taking opioids in a manner or dose other than prescribed or taking opioids for non-medical use. Abuse often starts as misuse of prescription opioids.

[2] For the purposes of this chapter, we use the term opioids to refer to prescription opioid pain relievers, such as hydrocodone or oxycodone, rather than illicit substances, such as heroin. SAMHSA reports that in 2017, 97.2 percent of an estimated 11.4 million people age 12 or older who misused opioids in the past year misused prescription opioids, and 2.8 percent of these people misused heroin only. Health care providers include physicians, dentists, and mid-level practitioners (e.g., nurse practitioners or physician assistants) who can be licensed, registered, or otherwise permitted to prescribe a controlled substance.

to opioid abuse and can lead to overdoses. Overdoses involving prescription opioids—hereafter referred to as opioids—were five times higher in 2017 than in 1999, accounting for about 17,000 deaths in 2017.[3]

Federal, state and local government agencies, drug manufacturers, communities, and others have attempted to address the potential for misuse and abuse by identifying or providing safe, secure, and convenient methods for disposing of unused, unneeded, or expired opioids. However, there is no federal law or regulation imposing requirements for how patients are to dispose of unused opioids.

The SUPPORT for Patients and Communities Act (SUPPORT Act) included a provision for us to review options for patients to dispose of unused opioids, including products intended to facilitate in-home disposal.[4] In this chapter we describe:

1. The federally recommended and other available methods patients may use to dispose of unused opioids, and
2. What is known about patients' use of these methods to dispose of unused opioids and examples of efforts to educate patients and providers about opioid disposal.

To describe the methods that federal agencies recommend patients use to dispose of unused opioids, we reviewed documentation and interviewed officials from the three federal agencies that have authorities related to the disposal of opioids—the Drug Enforcement Administration (DEA), the Food and Drug Administration (FDA), and the Environmental Protection Agency (EPA). We analyzed data from DEA as of April 2019 indicating the locations of permanent drug take-back collection sites in conjunction with data from the U.S. Census Bureau's population estimates through 2017. We used these data to estimate the percentage of the U.S. population living within varying distances of a permanent collection site.[5] For all data

[3] Centers for Disease Control and Prevention (CDC), *Prescription Opioid Data*, accessed June 13, 2019, https://www.cdc.gov/drugoverdose/data/prescribing.html.

[4] Pub. L. No. 115-271, § 3032(d),132 Stat. 3894 (2018).

[5] We analyzed the most recent DEA and U.S. Census Bureau data available at the time of our analysis. The U.S. Census Bureau's American Community Survey 5-year estimates are

used in these analyses, we reviewed related documentation and conducted electronic testing and, based on these steps, determined that the data were sufficiently reliable for our purposes. To describe other disposal methods, we reviewed documents and studies from vendors of three commercial in-home disposal products that patients can use to help them dispose of prescription and nonprescription medication in their home trash. We identified these products and documents through stakeholder interviews, a related study, a patent search using Google Patents, and a review of product websites.[6] Additionally, we conducted interviews with other stakeholders—including researchers, a representative from the AmerisourceBergen Foundation, and representatives from three companies that manufacture in-home drug disposal products.[7] We asked these stakeholders about the effectiveness of these other disposal methods at preventing misuse of opioids.[8]

To describe what is known about which methods patients use to dispose of unused opioids, we conducted interviews with stakeholders, such as the Association for Accessible Medicines and the American Medical Association (AMA), and reviewed results of SAMHSA's 2017

---

updated annually and are based on data collected continuously from a sample of households during the entire 60-month period. We used the 5-year estimates rather than 1-year estimates because they are based on larger sample sizes and thus are more reliable. To conduct this analysis, we calculated the distance between the central point of each zip code and the nearest DEA-registered permanent collection site. For some zip codes, depending upon whether their central point is located just within the distance threshold or just beyond it, a portion of their population may be unintentionally included in or excluded from the population subtotal and total, thus introducing a small degree of error in the percentage calculation. The radius of each distance category was not limited by state boundaries, and we chose these distance thresholds based on a review of available information on convenient distances for accessing pharmacies.

[6] Community Environmental Health Strategies LLC, *Medicine Disposal Products: An Overview of Products and Performance Questions,* (2019). Community Environmental Health Strategies is a consulting firm that prepared this chapter for the San Francisco Department of the Environment.

[7] We selected manufacturers of two products that are distributed in retail outlets and one newer product that has not been broadly distributed.

[8] The AmerisourceBergen Foundation is an independent not-for-profit charitable giving organization established by the AmerisourceBergen Corporation to support health-related causes that enrich the global community, including by supporting distribution of in-home drug disposal products to communities.

National Survey on Drug Use and Health.[9] We also conducted a literature review. Specifically, we performed a structured search of research databases— such as Scopus, ProQuest, ProQuest Dialog, and Harvard Think Tank— to identify literature published from January 1, 2009 through February 2019. In our search, we used a combination of terms such as "controlled substance," "disposal," "drug," and "prescription." These searches retrieved 846 results, of which 191 studies were selected by a librarian based on general relevancy for further review. We selected 25 studies based on the following criteria: if the study was published after January 1, 2014 and (1) presented findings that assessed the effectiveness of certain methods for disposing of opioids and other medications, (2) documented the quantity of unused opioids in the community, (3) examined how patients disposed of unused opioids, or (4) evaluated patient attitudes toward opioid disposal.[10] The findings from each individual study are limited by the studies' overall lack of national representation and small patient populations; however, taken together, we found that the methods and conclusions were sufficient for our purposes. To describe examples of efforts to educate patients and providers about opioid disposal, we interviewed officials from FDA and the AMA and reviewed relevant documentation from each.

We conducted this performance audit from December 2018 to September 2019 in accordance with generally accepted government auditing standards. Those standards require that we plan and perform the audit to obtain sufficient, appropriate evidence to provide a reasonable basis for our findings and conclusions based on our audit objectives. We believe that the evidence obtained provides a reasonable basis for our findings and conclusions based on our audit objectives.

---

[9] The National Survey on Drug Use and Health collects data through interviews with U.S. civilians who are not institutionalized. In the survey, respondents are asked about their drug use, among other things. Based on these responses, SAMHSA estimates results for the U.S. population. Results from the 2017 survey were the most recent data available at the time of our analysis.

[10] We selected studies published after January 1, 2014 because DEA's final rule governing disposal of controlled substances was released in 2014. See 79 Fed. Reg. 53,520, 53,548 (Sept. 9, 2014).

BACKGROUND

Opioids, such as hydrocodone and oxycodone, can be prescribed to treat both acute and chronic pain. Opioids can pose serious risks when they are misused. These risks include addiction, overdose, and death. As a result, opioids are classified as controlled substances, which means that their use and disposal are subject to additional oversight by DEA.[11]

Some studies suggest that the majority of patients who received prescriptions for opioids often do not use a large portion of the drugs dispensed. A study that surveyed U.S. adults who had received opioids found that approximately 60 percent of patients who were no longer using the medication had unused opioids.[12] Two studies reported that over one-half of patients did not use all of the opioids prescribed to them after surgery; these studies found that patients reported leaving 15 to 20 pills unused, representing 54 percent to 72 percent of the opioids they were prescribed.[13] Another study on patient opioid use after a cesarean section and thoracic surgery found that most patients, 83 percent and 71 percent respectively, used less than half of the total opioids they were prescribed.[14]

Federal Authorities

There is no federal law or regulation imposing requirements for how patients are to dispose of unused opioids. However, DEA, FDA, and EPA all have authorities and initiatives related to patient disposal of opioids.

---

[11] Controlled substances are regulated under the Controlled Substances Act, which is enforced by DEA. See Pub. L. No. 91-513, tit. III, 84 Stat. 1236, 1242-84 (1970) (codified, as amended, at 21 U.S.C. § 801 et seq.).

[12] A. Kennedy-Hendricks et al., "Medication Sharing, Storage, and Disposal Practices for Opioid Medications Among US Adults," *JAMA Internal Medicine*, vol. 176, no. 7 (2016): p. 1027-1029.

[13] M. V. Hill et al., "Wide Variation and Excessive Dosage of Opioid Prescriptions for Common General Surgical Procedures," *Annals of Surgery*, vol. 265, no. 4 (2017): p. 709- 714 and B. C. Maughan et al., "Unused Opioid Analgesics and Drug Disposal Following Outpatient Dental Surgery: A Randomized Control Trial," *Drug and Alcohol Dependence*, vol. 168 (2016): p. 328-334.

[14] K. Bartels et al., "Opioid Use and Storage Patterns by Patients after Hospital Discharge following Surgery," *PLoS ONE*, vol. 11, no. 1 (2016).

DEA

DEA regulations specify three take-back options that patients can opt to use to dispose of their unused controlled substances: take-back events, permanent collection sites, and mail-back programs. DEA hosts semi-annual events called National Prescription Drug Take-Back Days, where temporary collection sites are set up in locations such as police stations.[15] Advertisements encourage community participation in the events and educate the community on safe disposal of unused medications, including opioids. DEA also registers collectors and provides information to the public about the location of permanent collection sites for take-back, such as at local retail pharmacies or hospital pharmacies, and sets requirements for the provision of postage-paid envelopes that patients can use to mail unused drugs to a collector for destruction.[16]

DEA regulations establish a standard for the destruction of controlled substances that applies to DEA registrants, which can destroy opioids on patients' behalf.[17] DEA registrants include pharmaceutical companies that manufacture controlled substances, health care providers who prescribe them, and pharmacies that dispense them. The standard for destruction requires that controlled substances maintained or collected by DEA registrants be rendered non-retrievable. This means that the physical and chemical conditions of the controlled substance must be permanently altered, thereby rendering the controlled substance unavailable and unusable for all practical purposes.

---

[15] Federal, state, tribal, and local law enforcement may also collect unused controlled substances through other take-back events, mail-back programs, or collection receptacles located inside the law enforcement's premises. See 21 C.F.R. §§ 1317.35 and 1317.65 (2018).

[16] Under the Controlled Substances Act, all persons or entities that manufacture, distribute, or dispense controlled substances are required to register with DEA, unless specifically exempted. DEA regulates these entities to limit diversion and prevent abuse. DEA registrants must receive authorization from DEA to collect controlled substances for disposal. Authorized collectors may (1) receive and destroy mail-back packages; (2) install, manage, and maintain collection receptacles located at their collection locations; and (3) dispose of sealed inner liners from collection receptacles, including their contents. 21 C.F.R. § 1317.40(c) (2018).

[17] A patient who receives a prescription for a controlled substance is not a DEA registrant and therefore is not subject to this standard.

According to DEA, as of May 2019, the only method currently used to meet this standard is incineration, and DEA rulemaking states that DEA will not evaluate, review, or approve methods used to render a controlled substance non-retrievable.[18]

FDA

FDA has broad authority under the Federal Food, Drug, and Cosmetic Act to evaluate whether a drug is safe and effective and ensure the benefits of drugs outweigh the risks. FDA may require manufacturers to develop a risk evaluation and mitigation strategy (REMS) for drugs with serious safety risks, including the risk of abuse, to ensure that the benefits outweigh the risks.[19] Under one REMS, for example, manufacturers of opioids intended for outpatient use must make training available to health care providers involved in the treatment and monitoring of patients who receive opioids. The training must contain certain elements, including how providers should counsel patients and caregivers about the safe use and disposal of these opioids, among other things.

In October 2018, the SUPPORT Act authorized FDA to, at its discretion, require specific packaging or disposal systems as a part of certain drugs' REMS.[20] For drugs with a serious risk of overdose or abuse, FDA may require the drug to be made available for dispensing to certain patients with "safe disposal packaging" or a "safe disposal system" for purposes of rendering the drug non-retrievable in accordance with DEA regulations.[21] Before imposing these requirements, FDA must consider the potential burden on patient access to the drug and the health care delivery system.

---

[18] 79 Fed. Reg. 53,520, 53,548 (Sept. 9, 2014). DEA regulations do not specify a test for evaluating whether a method meets the non-retrievable standard.

[19] GAO has forthcoming work that examines risk evaluation and mitigation strategies.

[20] Pub. L. No. 115-271, § 3032(a),132 Stat. 3894 (2018) (codified at 21 U.S.C. § 355- 1(e)(4)).

[21] The SUPPORT Act also authorized FDA to require that certain drugs be made available for dispensing in unit dose packaging, packaging that provides a set duration, or another packaging system that FDA determines may mitigate serious risk of overdose or abuse. On May 31, 2019, FDA issued a notice in the Federal Register soliciting comments about unit dose packaging for opioids. 84 Fed. Reg. 25,283 (May 31, 2019).

As of May 2019, FDA had not imposed any REMS requirements using the new SUPPORT Act authority.

EPA

Under the Resource Conservation and Recovery Act (RCRA), EPA has authority to regulate the generation, transportation, treatment, storage, and disposal of hazardous waste, including certain discarded opioids.[22] However, hazardous waste pharmaceuticals generated by households are not regulated as hazardous waste even if the waste would otherwise be considered hazardous.[23] Opioids and other household waste pharmaceuticals collected through a take-back option are also exempt from most hazardous waste regulations, provided certain conditions are met.[24] Some states and localities have imposed additional requirements for pharmaceutical disposal, such as requirements for drug manufacturers to manage or fund the disposal of collected household pharmaceuticals.

---

[22] A waste is "hazardous" under RCRA if EPA has specifically listed it as such by regulation, or if it exhibits one of four hazardous characteristics (ignitability, corrosivity, reactivity, or toxicity). See 40 C.F.R. § 261.3(a)(2)(2018). EPA may authorize states to implement their own hazardous waste management programs in lieu of the federal program as long as, among other things, the state programs are at least equivalent to the federal program. Authorized states may implement regulations that are more stringent or broader in scope than the federal regulations. 42 U.S.C. § 6926(b).

[23] While a small percentage of pharmaceuticals discarded by households meet the definition of hazardous waste under RCRA, EPA regulations specify that solid waste generated by households, including pharmaceuticals, are not regulated as hazardous waste. 40 C.F.R. § 261.4(b)(1) (2018) and 84 Fed. Reg. 5,816, 5,941 (Feb. 22, 2019) (to be codified at 40 C.F.R. § 266.501(g)(7)). Household hazardous waste pharmaceuticals are allowed to be disposed of as municipal solid waste when discarded by individuals at their residences.

[24] To meet the conditional exemption, collected household hazardous waste pharmaceuticals must be: (1) managed in compliance with EPA's prohibition on discharging hazardous waste pharmaceuticals to a sewer system that passes through to a public-owned treatment works; (2) collected, transported, stored, and disposed of in compliance with all applicable DEA regulations for controlled substances; and (3) destroyed by a method DEA has publicly deemed in writing to meet the non-retrievable standard of destruction or combusted at one of five permitted types of hazardous waste combustors. 84 Fed. Reg. 5,816, 5,945 (Feb. 22, 2019) (to be codified at 40 C.F.R. § 266.506). If these conditions are not met, it is the entity collecting the pharmaceuticals, and not the consumer, that is subject to EPA's hazardous waste regulations.

FEDERAL AGENCIES RECOMMEND TAKE-BACK OPTIONS AS THE PREFERRED DISPOSAL METHOD

Federal Agencies Recommend Take-Back Options Whenever Feasible, Followed by Disposal Using the Toilet or Trash

According to DEA, FDA, and EPA, patients should use take-back options to dispose of unused opioids, whenever feasible. Only if take-back options are not feasible, FDA recommends flushing opioids on FDA's flush list down the toilet to remove them from the home as soon as possible.[25]

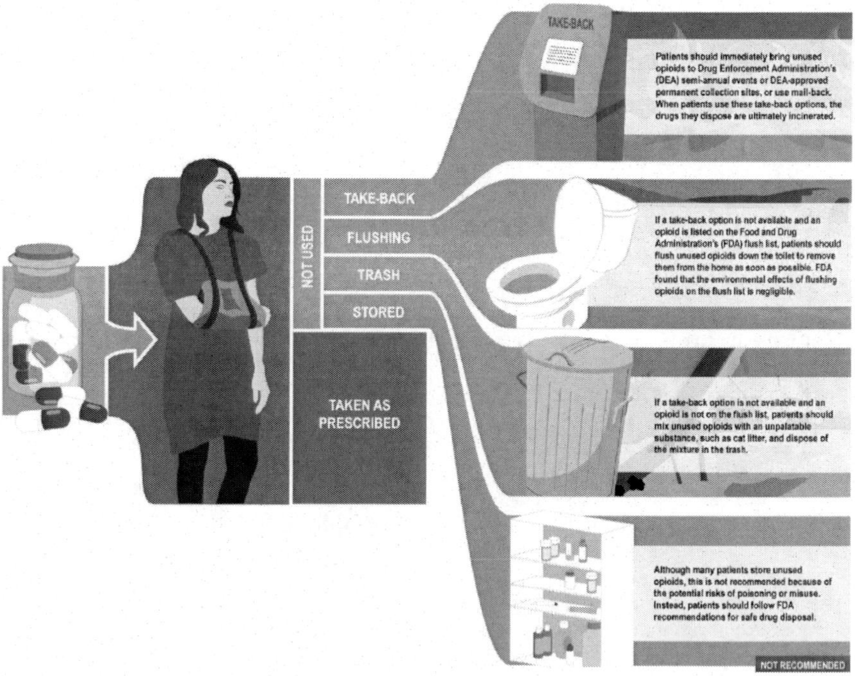

Source: GAO analysis of FDA documents. | GAO-19-650.

Figure 1. Patient Use and Food and Drug Administration's Recommendations for Disposal of Prescription Opioids.

---

[25] See *Environmental Health: Action Needed to Sustain Agencies' Collaboration on Pharmaceuticals in Drinking Water,* GAO-11-346 (Washington, D.C.: Aug. 8, 2011) for prior GAO work related to pharmaceuticals in drinking water.

For opioids not on the flush list, the agencies recommend placing the drugs in the household trash mixed with an unpalatable substance.[26] (See Figure 1). Officials from FDA said that the primary goal of these recommendations is to remove dangerous substances from the home as soon as possible to reduce accidental poisoning, which also may address issues related to intentional misuse. FDA officials explained that the agency has not measured the effects of its recommendations for disposing of opioids on opioid misuse, as of May 2019, because it is difficult to establish a causal link between the recommendations and any reductions in misuse.

Take-Back Options

DEA, FDA, and EPA recommend using a take-back option as the preferred method for patients to dispose of unused prescription opioids. Under this method, patients can bring unused opioids to DEA's semi-annual take-back events or to DEA-registered permanent collection sites, or use mail-back to deliver opioids to a DEA-registered collector for destruction. When patients use these take-back options, the drugs they dispose of are ultimately incinerated, which is the only method that DEA officials said is known to render the drugs non-retrievable, that is, permanently and irreversibly destroyed.

Our analysis of DEA and U.S. Census Bureau data shows that as of April 2019, 71 percent of the country's population lived less than 5 miles from a permanent collection site, and in 42 states, at least half of the population lived within 5 miles of a site. (See Figure 2). This number has increased since our April 2017 report, when we found that about half of the country's population lived less than 5 miles away from a site.[27]

---

[26] FDA officials reported that these drug disposal recommendations were first developed by the Office of the National Drug Control Policy in 2007.

[27] See GAO, *Preventing Drug Abuse: Low Participation by Pharmacies and Other Entities as Voluntary Collectors of Unused Prescription Drugs,* GAO-18-25 (Washington, D.C.: Oct. 12, 2017). Our analysis was limited to permanent DEA-registered collection sites that use receptacles to collect unused prescription drugs from the public and does not include disposal options provided by law enforcement agencies, which do not need to register with DEA to collect controlled substances.

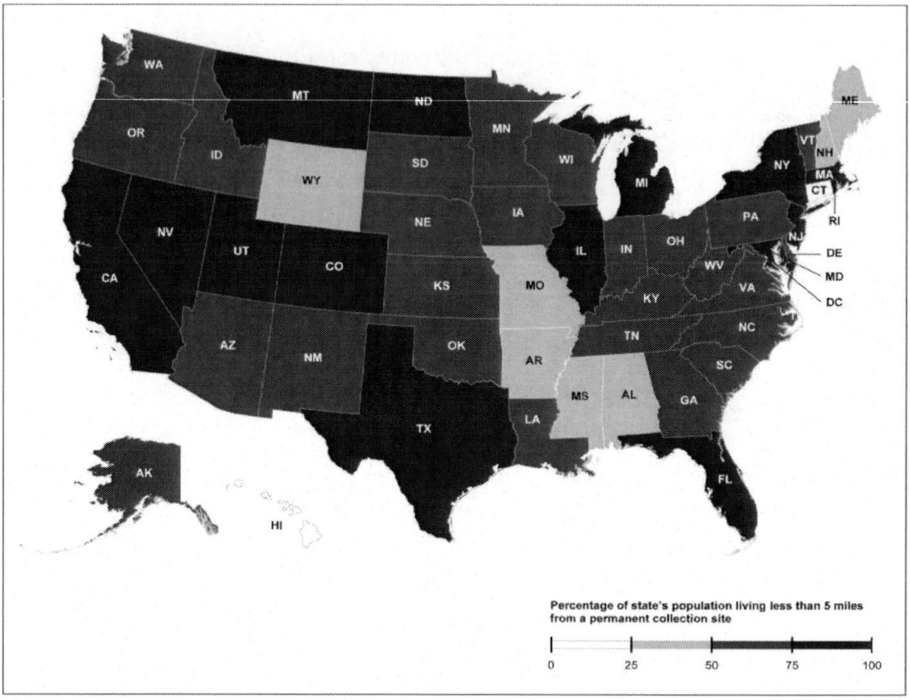

Source: GAO analysis of Drug Administration and U.S. Census Bureau data; Map Resources (map). | GAO-19-650.

Note: We analyzed April 2019 data from DEA about the locations of non-law enforcement entities that are authorized to install receptacles to collect controlled substances for disposal by the general public. We also used 2017 U.S. Census Bureau population estimates to estimate, by zip code, the portion of the population within certain distances of a permanent collection site.

Figure 2. Estimated Percentage of Population Living Less Than 5 Miles From a Drug Enforcement Administration (DEA)- Registered Drug Take-Back Permanent Collection Site, by State, April 2019.

Our analysis also shows that 90 percent of the population lived within 15 miles of a site, though in rural areas only 57 percent lived within 15 miles. In addition, two studies found that patients were willing to bring unused opioids to a take-back location as long as it was located within 5 to 8 miles of their home address.[28]

[28] K. I. Stoddard et al., "Investigating Research Gaps of Pharmaceutical Take-Back Events: An Analysis of Take-Back Program Participants' Socioeconomic, Demographic, and

Flushing

If take-back options are not feasible, FDA recommends flushing the opioids on its flush list down the toilet, because a single dose can be fatal to a child or a pet. Flushing is a permanent way to remove opioids from the home.[29] FDA confirmed that as of June 2019, 11 of 14 drugs on the flush list are opioids, which represents about three-quarters of the approved opioid active ingredients intended for outpatient use (see sidebar). Some portion of drugs that are flushed down the toilet ultimately enter surface and wastewater streams.

Food and Drug Administration's Flush List, as of May 2019

- Benzhydrocodone/Acetaminophen
- Buprenorphine
- Fentanyl
- Diazepam*
- Hydrocodone
- Hydromorphone
- Meperidine
- Methadone
- Methylphenidate*
- Morphine
- Oxycodone
- Oxymorphone
- Tapentadol
- Sodium Oxybate*

*These drugs are not opioids.

Source: Food and Drug Administration | GAO-19-650.

Geographic Characteristics and the Public Health Benefits of Take-Back Programs," *Environmental Management*, vol. 59 (2017): p. 871-884 and M. A. Kozak, "A Needs Assessment of Unused and Expired Medication Disposal Practices: A Study From The Medication Safety Research Network of Indiana," *Research in Social and Administrative Pharmacy*, vol. 12 (2016): p. 336-340.

[29] The flush list does not include antibiotics and hormones, which have known detrimental environmental effects. See https://www.fda.gov/drugs/safe-disposal-medicines/disposal-unused-medicines-what-youshould-know (accessed June 4, 2019). Opioids have been detected in wastewater samples in the US, Canada, Europe, South America, and Asia. See Campos-Manas et al, "Trends in Environmental Analytical Chemistry," (2018).

However, a 2017 FDA study on the environmental impact of drugs listed on the flush list concluded that flushing these opioids has negligible effects on the environment and human health, particularly relative to the amount of opioids that are excreted after taking them as prescribed, because not all of the drug is metabolized.[30] (See text box for a summary of the effects of disposal options on the environment).

Environmental Effects of Disposal Options

The environmental impact of opioid disposal depends on the method used—take-back options, flushing, or trash. According to Environmental Protection Agency (EPA) and Drug Enforcement Agency (DEA) officials, disposal of drugs through take-back options results in disposal by permitted incineration, which fully destroys the active form of the drugs. EPA officials told us that flushing or placing opioids in the trash can introduce active opioids into wastewater streams, groundwater, and surface waters.

Incineration of Drugs from Take-Back Options. Opioids disposed of using take-back options are destroyed by incineration, which, according to DEA officials, is the only method currently used to meet its non-retrievable standard for destruction. EPA officials told us that based on data from DEA, the amount of household pharmaceutical waste gathered and incinerated during DEA's semi-annual take-back events is small compared to the total amount of waste one incinerator burns on an average day. EPA officials recommended take-back options as the preferred method of opioid disposal.

Flushing. Opioids enter the water supply when excreted by patients who take opioids as prescribed and when patients intentionally flush unused opioids down the toilet. EPA officials told us that most wastewater treatment facilities are not designed to eliminate opioids from wastewater streams. Further, measureable concentrations of opioids have been reported in surface and ground water sources around the world.

Trash. Disposal of unused opioids in the trash often introduces opioids into landfills. Studies in scientific literature show that pharmaceutical ingredients have been observed in the water that passes through landfills, called leachate. Similar to opioids that are flushed, opioids in landfill leachate can end up in wastewater streams and other water sources, according to EPA officials.

Source: GAO analysis of information from EPA and DEA | GAO-19-650.

[30] U. Khan et al., "Risks Associated With the Environmental Release of Pharmaceuticals on the U.S. Food and Drug Administration 'Flush List'," *Science of the Total Environment*, vol. 609 (2017). This study did not examine the human and environmental impacts of flushing drugs other than those on FDA's flush list.

Household Trash

If an opioid is not on the FDA flush list and a take-back option is not feasible, the agencies direct patients to take a series of steps to dispose of their opioids in household trash by:

1. mixing the drugs in an unpalatable substance such as dirt, cat litter, or used coffee grounds,
2. placing the mixture in a sealed container or plastic bag, and
3. throwing the container in the trash.

An EPA official said that mixing the drugs with an unpalatable substance is meant to deter misusers from searching through the trash to retrieve the drugs. Disposal of opioids in the trash—either with an unpalatable substance or in-home disposal product—removes them from the home, but this option may not be permanent and the drugs still may be available for misuse. Drugs that are disposed in the trash ultimately are introduced to landfills, where they can escape landfill containment and enter wastewater streams or ground water sources.

FDA Has Not Evaluated Commercial Disposal Methods

FDA's website notes the availability of commercial products for disposing of unused opioids and other drugs in the home.[31] FDA officials stated that, as of May 2019, the agency had not evaluated the effectiveness of these products or made any recommendations related to their use, but they are aware that patients may opt to use these products.[32] These products, known as in-home disposal products, are proprietary substances that patients can mix with their unused drugs, including opioids, before

---

[31] See https://www.fda.gov/drugs/safe-disposal-medicines/disposal-unused-medicines-what-you-should-know (accessed June 4, 2019).

[32] The SUPPORT Act allows FDA to require as part of a REMS that certain drugs be dispensed with safe disposal packaging or a safe disposal system for purposes of rendering the drug non-retrievable in accordance with DEA regulations. Pub. L. No. 115- 271, § 3032(a),132 Stat. 3894 (2018) (codified at 21 U.S.C. § 355-1(e)(4)).

disposing of them in the trash. In-home disposal product vendors told us they sell or donate their products to pharmacies, local law enforcement, and community groups, which then distribute them to patients.[33] A representative from a group that distributes these products, the AmerisourceBergen Foundation, noted that in-home disposal products may be a convenient option for patients for whom take-back options are not feasible, and marketing materials from a product vendor instruct patients to use their product if a take-back option is not available. Vendors indicate that their products can prevent misuse of opioids by rendering drugs non-retrievable at home and by motivating patients to dispose of unused opioids. According to DEA officials, rendering opioids non-retrievable by using an in-home disposal product is challenging, because the drugs have a variety of chemical and physical properties and potencies. Furthermore, according to DEA officials, a lethal dose of fentanyl can be as low as 250 micrograms in adults—and lower in children—underscoring the importance of effective disposal.

Some vendors have presented evaluations of their commercial products. A recent comprehensive review of eight in-home disposal products raised concerns about the credibility of vendors' evaluations and concluded that additional independent laboratory analysis is needed to fully examine product performance and assess how well these products achieve stated goals.[34] Our review of evaluations from three vendors found that the studies contained some inconsistencies and gaps in the evaluation methods used, raising questions about the studies' conclusions that the products are effective for disposing of opioids.

- In some cases, studies included detailed, but inconsistent, methods. For example, in four studies about one product, the researchers concluded that the product deactivated most of an opioid dissolved

---

[33] All three product vendors we spoke with said that all or nearly all of their sales are to organizations that distribute products to patients rather than to patients themselves. For example, one vendor representative said that the in-home disposal product is available to patients for free at approximately 40 percent of all chain drugstores nationwide.

[34] Community Environmental Health Strategies LLC, *Medicine Disposal Products: An Overview of Products and Performance Questions,* (2019).

in water. However, one of the earlier studies reported that whole pills did not dissolve in water, which could impact the results, but later studies did not include similar data.

- In other cases, companies' evaluations were summaries of results that did not provide enough information to independently verify or assess whether the products deactivate opioids and prevent misuse. For example, one company's research documents presented images of a mixture as evidence that the drugs had degraded, rather than results of a test measuring if drugs were still detectable.
- In addition, the studies included little information about the products' effectiveness at treating mixtures of multiple drugs at the same time, a scenario that stakeholders have referred to as "real world" use testing.

Few Patients Use Federally Recommended Opioid Disposal Methods; FDA and Others Have Taken Steps to Educate the Public

Few Patients Use Federally Recommended Methods to Dispose of Unused Opioids

Disposal methods—when patients use them promptly—remove unused opioids from the home and therefore can be effective at reducing opioid misuse. FDA officials said that the federally recommended methods for disposing unused opioids are intended to remove these substances from the home as soon as possible, and stated that as long as individuals dispose of opioids promptly rather than storing them, then FDA has achieved its goal.

However, the studies we reviewed suggest that most patients do not dispose of unused opioids using a federally recommended method. Specifically, three studies examined how patients disposed of unused opioids and found that between 12 percent and 41 percent of patients disposed of them using a federally recommended method.[35] For example, one of the studies found that of 570 survey respondents who had unused opioids, 12 percent of respondents reported using a take-back option, 14 percent reported that they flushed them down the toilet, and 6 percent reported that they threw them in the trash after mixing with an unpalatable substance.[36]

Other studies we reviewed show that take-back options are often used to dispose of drugs other than opioids. Two studies found that less than 10 percent of the catalogued drugs brought to DEA take-back days were controlled substances, which included opioids, while another study weighed drugs brought to take-back events and permanent collection sites and reported less than 3 percent were controlled substances, including opioids.[37] The same study found that annually, controlled substances disposed of at take-back events and permanent collection sites accounted for about 0.3 percent of those dispensed in the area, and concluded that take-back events may have a minimal impact on reducing the availability of unused opioids for misuse.[38]

---

[35] M. V. Hill et al., "Wide Variation and Excessive Dosage of Opioid Prescriptions for Common General Surgical Procedures," 709-714 and A. Kennedy-Hendricks et al., "Medication Sharing, Storage, and Disposal Practices for Opioid Medications Among US Adults," 1027-1029 and M.J. Sabatino et. al., "Excess Opioid Medication and Variation in Prescribing Patterns Following Common Orthopaedic Procedures," *Journal of Bone and Joint Surgery*, vol. 100-A, no. 3 (2018): p. 180-188.

[36] Kennedy-Hendricks et al., "Medication Sharing, Storage, and Disposal Practices for Opioid Medications Among US Adults," 1027-1029.

[37] DEA regulations prohibit authorized collectors from opening and cataloging the contents of permanent collection receptacles. 21 C.F.R. § 1317.75(c) (2018). Evaluations of the use and contents of collection receptacles are limited to receptacles maintained by law enforcement agencies, which are not subject to this prohibition. We identified three studies conducted in conjunction with law enforcement agencies that quantified the amount of opioids collected via collection receptacles: C. S. Ma et al., "Drug Take Back in Hawai'i: Partnership Between the University of Hawai'I Hilo College of Pharmacy and the Narcotics Enforcement Division," *Journal of Medicine and Public Health*, vol. 73, no. 1 (2014): p. 26- 30 and H. Stewart et al., "Inside Maine's Medicine Cabinet: Findings From Drug Enforcement Administration's Medication Take-back Events," *American Journal of Public Health*, vol. 105, no. 1 (2015): p. e65-e71 and K. L. Egan et al., "From Dispensed to Disposed: Evaluating the Effectiveness of Disposal Programs Through a Comparison with Prescription Drug Monitoring Program Data," *The American Journal of Drug and Alcohol Abuse*, vol. 43, no. 1 (2017): p. 69-77.

[38] K. L. Egan et al., "From Dispensed to Disposed," 69-77.

Studies indicate that patients who receive an in-home disposal product may be more likely to dispose of unused opioids, but they may also be less likely to use federally recommended options like take-back or flushing. Two studies in our review found that patients who receive an in-home disposal product have reported that they are more likely to dispose of unused opioids than those who did not receive the product.[39] Use of in-home disposal products—which may not be effective at permanently destroying drugs—may deter patients from using federally recommended options, like take-back, that have been proven effective. For example, one of these studies found that only one of the 70 patients who received an in-home disposal product used a take-back option for disposal, despite the study taking place in a state where we estimated that 77 percent of the population lived less than 5 miles from a permanent collection site.

Studies indicate that patients are often unaware of federally recommended disposal options. Three of the 25 studies we reviewed suggest that many patients were not aware of federally recommended methods for disposing of opioids.[40] For example, a study of cancer patients who received opioid prescriptions reported that more than three-quarters of these patients were unaware of proper opioid disposal methods.[41] Another 2016 study of 1,032 patients found that nearly half of the respondents did not recall receiving information on proper disposal from pharmacists, medication packaging, or media outlets.[42]

---

[39] C. M. Brummett, R. Steiger, M. Engelsbe, et. al., "Effect of an Activated Charcoal Bag on Disposal of Unused Opioids After an Outpatient Surgical Procedure: A Randomized Clinical Trial," *JAMA Surgery,* (2019) and A. E. Lawrence, A.. J. Carsel, K. L. Leonhardt et al., "Effect of Drug Disposal Bag Provision on Proper Disposal of Unused Opioids by Families of Pediatric Surgical Patients: A Randomized Clinical Trial,"*JAMA Pediatrics,* (Published online June 24, 2019).

[40] Kozak et al., "A Needs Assessment of Unused and Expired Medication Disposal Practices," 336-340 and Kennedy-Hendricks et al., "Medication Sharing, Storage, and Disposal Practices for Opioid Medications Among US Adults," 1027-1029 and J. Silvestre et al., "Frequency of Unsafe Storage, Use, and Disposal Practices of Opioids Among Cancer Patients Presenting to the Emergency Department," *Palliative and Supportive Care*, vol. 15 (2017): p. 638-643.

[41] J. Silvestre et al., "Frequency of Unsafe Storage, Use, and Disposal Practices of Opioids Among Cancer Patients Presenting to the Emergency Department," 638-643.

[42] Kennedy-Hendricks et al., "Medication Sharing, Storage, and Disposal Practices for Opioid Medications Among US Adults," 1027-1029.

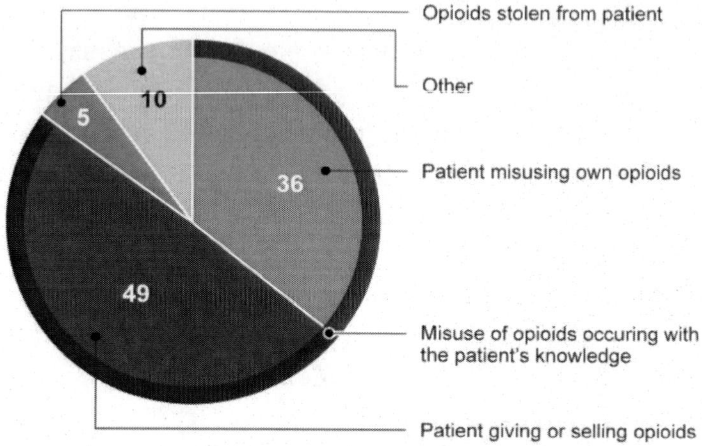

Source: GAO analysis of Substance Abuse and Mental Health Services Administration data. | GAO-19-650.

Note: "Other" sources for misused opioids include approximately 6 percent of misusers who bought the opioids from a drug dealer or other stranger and about 5 percent who obtained them some other way. These data are from the 2017 National Survey on Drug Use and Health, a nationally representative survey that asks people about their drug use within the past year, among other things, and includes a question about the source of the last opioids that a respondent misused. Misuse occurs when a person uses a drug in a way not intended by the prescriber, such as a patient taking a prescribed medicine to relieve pain other than the pain for which the drug was prescribed or taking a prescription intended for another person.

Figure 3. Ways People Obtained Opioids for Misuse in 2017 (percent).

Studies also indicate that patients choose not to dispose of unused opioids, and that they knowingly participate in the majority of opioid misuse. Five of the studies we reviewed found that between one-quarter and three-quarters of patients stored unused opioids for future use or had misplaced their unused opioids.[43] For example, one of these studies found

[43] Hill et al., "Wide Variation and Excessive Dosage of Opioid Prescriptions for Common General Surgical Procedures," 709-714; Kennedy-Hendricks et al., "Medication Sharing, Storage, and Disposal Practices for Opioid Medications Among US Adults," 1027-1029; D. D. Maeng et. al., "Unused Medications and Disposal Patterns at Home: Findings From a Medicare Patient Survey and Claims Data," *Journal of the American Pharmacists Association*, vol. 56 (2016): p. 41-46; and M.J. Sabatino et. al., "Excess Opioid Medication

that 49 percent of survey respondents kept or planned to keep unused opioids for future use, and 14 percent were likely to let a family member use their opioid medications in the future.[44] Federal data about the sources of misused opioids indicate that patients are complicit with most misuse. SAMHSA estimates that 5 percent of people nationwide who misused opioids in 2017 took these drugs from someone else without asking. In contrast, SAMHSA estimates that 85 percent of opioid misuse occurs with the patient's knowledge or active participation, either through the patient misusing his or her own prescription by taking the drug for pain other than for which it was prescribed or by giving or selling the prescribed opioids to another person (See Figure 3).[45]

FDA and Others Have Taken Steps to Educate Patients and Providers about Appropriate Opioid Disposal

To motivate patients to use federally recommended methods to dispose of unused opioids, FDA and some physician organizations have created educational materials on safe disposal methods. For example, FDA launched a public awareness campaign called "Remove the Risk" on April 25, 2019—complete with educational materials such as public service announcements, social media posts, fact sheets, and other web-based content.[46] AMA representatives reported that the AMA has provided physicians with educational material on drug disposal and prescribing. Specifically, AMA representatives told us that the association has compiled a two-page document for physicians containing information about drug disposal, links to DEA information on nearby permanent collection sites and take-back events, and FDA guidance on safe disposal of medications. This document included recommendations for physicians

and Variation in Prescribing Patterns Following Common Orthopaedic Procedures," 180-188.

[44] Kennedy-Hendricks et al., "Medication Sharing, Storage, and Disposal Practices for Opioid Medications Among US Adults," 1027-1029.

[45] SAMHSA, *Key Substance Use and Mental Health Indicators.*

[46] See https://www.fda.gov/drugs/ensuring-safe-use-medicine/safe-opioid-disposal-remove-risk-outreach-toolkit (accessed June 11, 2019).

to talk to patients about safe use of prescription opioids, remind patients to store their medications in a safe place out of reach from children, and have a conversation with patients about the most appropriate ways to dispose of expired, unwanted, or unused opioids.

The AmerisourceBergen Foundation has also partnered with communities to promote safe opioid disposal by providing education about take-back options and commercial in-home disposal products to patients. A representative from the Foundation explained that its Safe Disposal Support Program provides non-profit organizations or municipalities with commercial in-home disposal products, which then can be distributed free of charge to other organizations, individuals, or households. It also recommends that patients use take-back options when available. The representative said that organizations are to demonstrate to patients how these products work either through a brief in-person demonstration at an event or through a video. According to the representative, these products and demonstrations help people reflect on what is in their home and needs to be disposed of, either using a product or a take-back option.

Despite such efforts, little is known about the extent to which stakeholders' efforts to educate the public are effective in increasing use of federally recommended disposal methods. FDA officials said that they are not aware of the extent to which providers are familiar with all disposal methods or the extent to which providers discuss the importance of proper disposal with patients. As part of FDA's REMS requirements for outpatient opioids, manufacturers must make training available to health care providers involved in the treatment and monitoring of patients who receive opioids, which includes information about the need to communicate with patients about disposal of unused drugs. FDA officials said that opioid manufacturers must assess the effectiveness of their REMS, including an assessment of prescribers', other health care providers including pharmacists', and patients' understanding of the key risk messages conveyed through the educational materials. FDA expects to receive the next REMS assessment with the results of these analyses in 2020. The AMA has not been able to measure the effects of its recommendations, but provided anecdotal feedback from its members that many physicians do not consistently speak to their patients about disposal.

FDA officials and AMA representatives indicated that in addition to educating patients on opioid disposal methods, focusing efforts on reducing the amount of unused opioids would be an effective approach for reducing misuse and abuse. For example, FDA officials said that adding packaging configurations that contain smaller quantities of certain opioids could help prescribers to more carefully consider the amount of opioid pain medication they prescribe.[47] This in turn may reduce the number of unused opioids available in the home that could be inappropriately accessed by family members or visitors, and could potentially reduce the risk for misuse and abuse. Representatives from the AMA explained that it and other organizations are working to provide opioid prescribing resources and guidance to help physicians effectively manage patients' pain, which representatives said will reduce the number of unused opioids available for misuse.[48] FDA officials and a researcher also noted that dispensing opioids in packaging that makes it easy to count the number of unused pills may help patients identify intentional misuse.

AGENCY COMMENTS

The FDA and EPA provided technical comments on a draft of this chapter, which we incorporated as appropriate; the DEA did not have comments.

---

[47] On May 31, 2019, FDA issued a notice in the Federal Register soliciting comments about unit-dose packaging for opioids. 84 Fed. Reg. 25,283 (May 31, 2019).

[48] For example, CDC developed and published the *CDC Guideline for Prescribing Opioids for Chronic Pain* to provide recommendations for the prescribing of opioid pain medication for patients 18 and older in primary care settings. AMA representatives cautioned, however, that opioid restriction policies have had unintended negative consequences on substance use and pain care. Representatives from the AMA explained that it and other organizations also provide resources and guidance to help physicians effectively screen and refer patients for substance use disorders.

We are sending copies of this chapter to the appropriate congressional committees, the Secretary of Health and Human Services, the Administrator of the DEA, the Administrator of the EPA, and other interested parties.

James Cosgrove
Director, Health Care.

In: Prescription Drugs
Editor: Karen Sue McKinney
ISBN: 978-1-53617-288-1

Chapter 4

PRESCRIPTION DRUG USE IN THE UNITED STATES, 2015–2016*

Crescent B. Martin, Craig M. Hales, Qiuping Gu and Cynthia L. Ogden

INTRODUCTION

Monitoring prescription drug use patterns at the population level [1] can inform research and clinical practice. These patterns may shift over time in response to changing health needs, updated clinical guidelines [2], policy changes, and other factors [1, 3]. The percentage of the U.S. population that used one or more prescription drugs increased from 1999–2000 through 2007–2008 [4]. This chapter describes prescription drug use by age, sex, and race and Hispanic origin in 2015–2016 and trends over the preceding decade.

* This is an edited, reformatted and augmented version of a U.S. Department of Health and Human Services, Centers for Disease Control and Prevention, National Center for Health Statistics, No. 334, dated May 2019.

KEY FINDINGS

Data from the National Health and Nutrition Examination Survey

- In 2015–2016, 45.8% of the U.S. population used prescription drugs in the past 30 days.
- Prescription drug use increased with age, from 18.0% of children under age 12 years to 85.0% of adults aged 60 and over.
- Prescription drug use was highest among non-Hispanic white persons followed by non-Hispanic black persons, and lowest among non-Hispanic Asian and Hispanic persons.
- The most commonly used types of drugs included bronchodilators for ages 0–11 years, central nervous system stimulants for ages 12–19, antidepressants for ages 20–59, and lipid-lowering drugs for ages 60 and over.
- The percentage of the U.S. population that used prescription drugs decreased over the preceding decade.

WHAT PERCENTAGE OF THE U.S. POPULATION USED ONE OR MORE PRESCRIPTION DRUGS IN THE PAST 30 DAYS IN 2015–2016, AND DID USE DIFFER BY AGE AND SEX?

In 2015–2016, 45.8% of the U.S. population used one or more prescription drugs in the past 30 days (Figure 1). Prescription drug use increased with age, overall and among males and females.

Overall, 18.0% of children aged 0–11 years, 27.0% of adolescents aged 12–19, 46.7% of adults aged 20–59, and 85.0% of adults aged 60 and over used prescription drugs in the past 30 days.

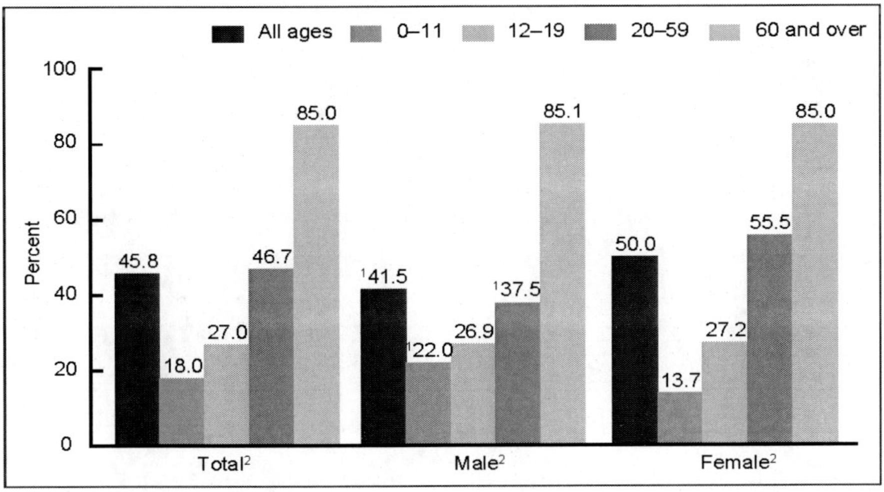

[1] Significantly different from females.

[2] Significant increasing trend with age.

Notes: Estimates for all ages are age adjusted by the direct method to the 2000 projected U.S. population using age groups 0–11, 12–19, 20–59, and 60 and over. Crude estimates are 48.1% for total, 43.0% for male, and 53.1% for female. Access data table for Figure 1 at: https://www.cdc.gov/nchs/data/databriefs/db334_tables-508.pdf#1.

Source: NCHS, National Health and Nutrition Examination Survey, 2015–2016.

Figure 1. Use of one or more prescription drugs in the past 30 days, by age (years) and sex: United States, 2015–2016.

Prescription drug use was lower among males (41.5%) than females (50.0%), although the pattern differed by age. Among children aged 0–11 years, prescription drug use was higher among boys (22.0%) than girls (13.7%), while among adults aged 20–59, prescription drug use was lower among men (37.5%) than women (55.5%). No significant differences by sex were observed among adolescents aged 12–19 or adults aged 60 and over.

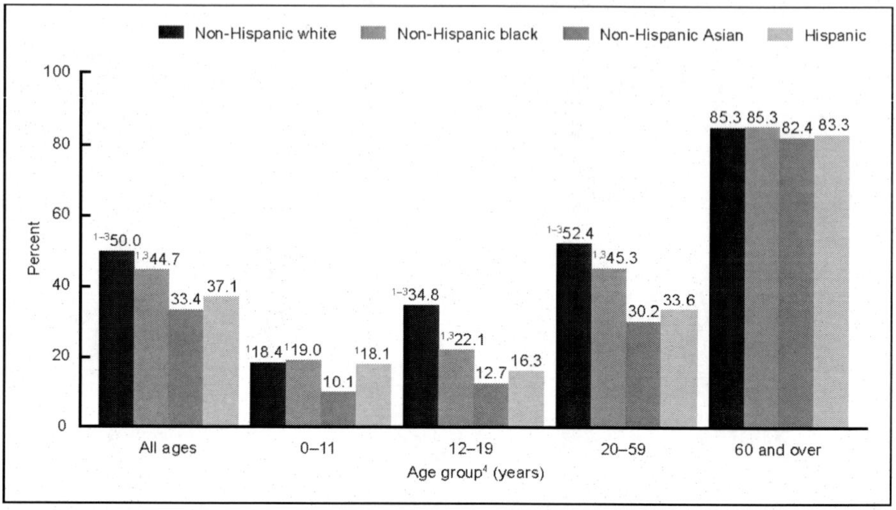

[1] Significantly different from non-Hispanic Asian persons.

[2] Significantly different from non-Hispanic black persons.

[3] Significantly different from Hispanic persons.

[4] Significant increasing trend with age.

Notes: Estimates for all ages were age adjusted by the direct method to the 2000 projected U.S. population using age groups 0–11, 12–19, 20–59, and 60 and over. Access data table for Figure 2 at: https://www.cdc.gov/nchs/data/databriefs/db334_tables-508.pdf#2.

Source: NCHS, National Health and Nutrition Examination Survey, 2015–2016.

Figure 2. Use of one or more prescription drugs in the past 30 days, by age and race and Hispanic origin: United States, 2015–2016.

Did Prescription Drug Use in the Past 30 Days Differ by Age and Race and Hispanic Origin in 2015–2016?

Overall, prescription drug use was higher among non-Hispanic white (50.0%) persons compared with non-Hispanic black (44.7%), Hispanic (37.1%), and non-Hispanic Asian (33.4%) persons (Figure 2). Prescription drug use was also higher among non-Hispanic black persons compared with non-Hispanic Asian and Hispanic persons. The patterns among adolescents aged 12–19 and adults aged 20–59 were similar to the overall pattern. Among adolescents, 34.8% of non-Hispanic white, 22.1% of non-Hispanic black, 12.7% of non-Hispanic Asian, and 16.3% of Hispanic adolescents used prescription drugs. Among adults aged 20–59, 52.4% of non-Hispanic white, 45.3% of non-Hispanic black, 30.2% of non-Hispanic Asian, and 33.6% of Hispanic adults used prescription drugs.

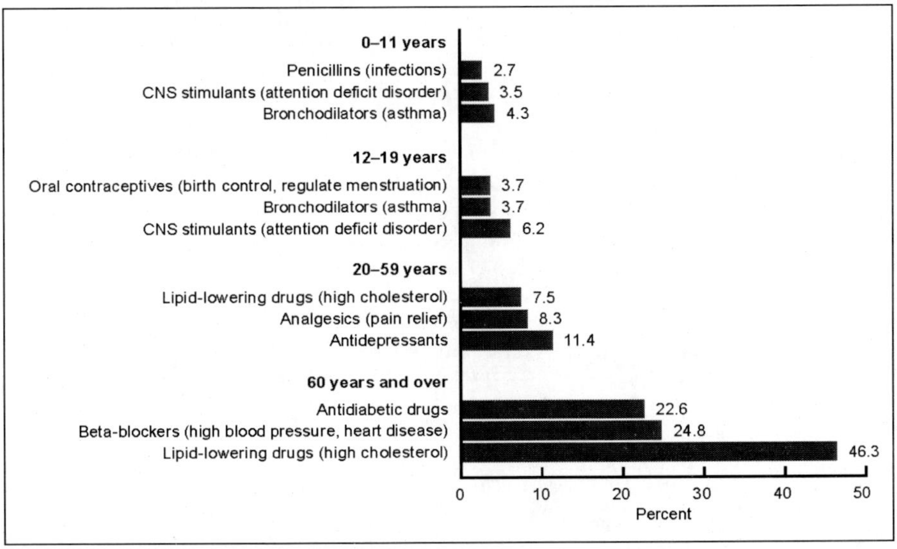

Notes: The primary indication for use of the drug type is in parentheses. Other drug types may also be used for the same indications as those shown. CNS is central nervous system. Oral contraceptives were used by 7.5% of girls aged 12–19. Access data table for Figure 3 at: https://www.cdc.gov/nchs/data/databriefs/db334_tables-508.pdf#3.

Source: NCHS, National Health and Nutrition Examination Survey, 2015–2016.

Figure 3. Use of the most commonly used prescription drug types in the past 30 days, by age group: United States, 2015–2016.

Among children aged 0–11 years, a lower percentage of non-Hispanic Asian children (10.1%) used prescription drugs compared with non-Hispanic white (18.4%), non-Hispanic black (19.0%), and Hispanic (18.1%) children. Among adults aged 60 and over, there were no differences between race and Hispanic-origin groups in the use of one or more prescription drugs.

For all race and Hispanic-origin groups, use of prescription drugs increased with age.

WHAT WERE THE MOST COMMONLY USED TYPES OF PRESCRIPTION DRUGS IN 2015–2016?

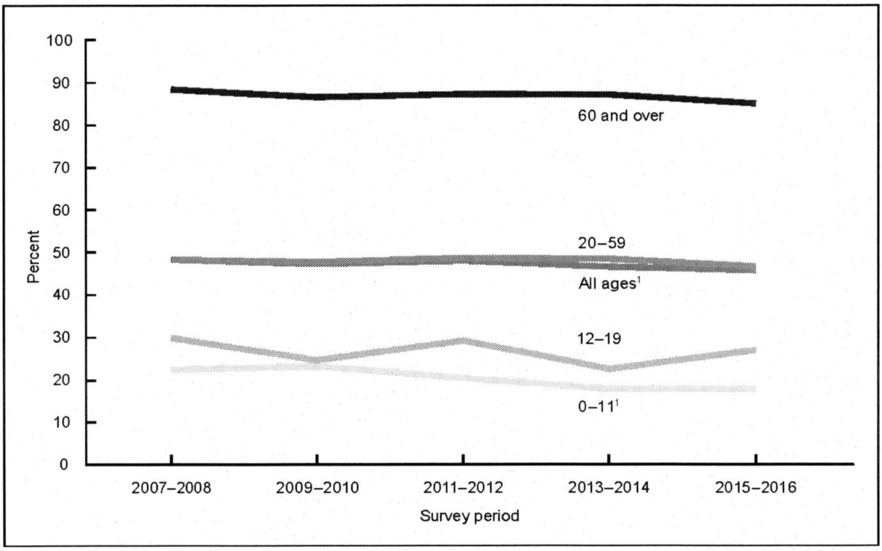

[1] Significant decreasing linear trend from 2007–2008 through 2015–2016.

Notes: Estimates for all ages are age adjusted by the direct method to the 2000 projected U.S. population using age groups 0–11, 12–19, 20–59, and 60 and over. Access data table for Figure 4 at: https://www.cdc.gov/nchs/data/databriefs/db334_tables-508.pdf#4.

Source: NCHS, National Health and Nutrition Examination Surveys, 2007–2016.

Figure 4. Trends in use of one or more prescription drugs in the past 30 days, by age (years): United States, 2007–2016.

The top three types of prescription drugs used by the U.S. population during 2015–2016 varied by age (Figure 3). The most commonly used prescription drug types in the past 30 days were bronchodilators for children aged 0–11 years (used by 4.3% of children), central nervous system stimulants for adolescents aged 12–19 (6.2%), antidepressants for adults aged 20–59 (11.4%), and lipid-lowering drugs for adults aged 60 and over (46.3%).

HAVE TRENDS IN PRESCRIPTION DRUG USE CHANGED OVER THE PRECEDING 10 YEARS?

Prescription drug use decreased among the U.S. population from 48.3% in 2007–2008 to 45.8% in 2015–2016 (Figure 4). Prescription drug use also decreased among children aged 0–11 years, from 22.4% in 2007–2008 to 18.0% in 2015–2016. The observed declines in prescription drug use among adults aged 20–59 and adults aged 60 and over were not statistically significant, and there was no significant trend among adolescents aged 12–19.

SUMMARY

During 2015–2016, almost one-half of the U.S. population used one or more prescription drugs in the past 30 days (45.8%). Prescription drug use increased with age, and a higher percentage of females (50.0%) than males (41.5%) used prescription drugs, but the pattern varied by age. Prescription drug use was higher in males among children aged 0–11 years but higher in females among adults aged 20–59, while there were no differences by sex among adolescents aged 12–19 or adults aged 60 and over. Patterns across race and Hispanic-origin groups also varied by age. Among adults aged 60 and over, no significant differences were observed among race and Hispanic-origin groups.

The most commonly used types of prescription drugs included bronchodilators for children aged 0–11 years, central nervous system stimulants for adolescents aged 12–19, antidepressants for adults aged 20–59, and lipid-lowering drugs for adults aged 60 and over. From 2007–2008 through 2015–2016, prescription drug use decreased for the overall population and for children aged 0–11 years.

Monitoring the use of prescription drugs may describe aspects of the health of the U.S. population. Differences in the most commonly used prescription drug types by age group illustrate differences in the prevalence of health conditions at various stages of life. Changing trends in prescription drug use over time may be influenced by changing disease prevalence and diagnosis [5, 6], expanded treatment recommendations [2, 7], and decline in the use of inappropriate or ineffective therapies [8, 9].

DEFINITIONS

Prescription Drug Use

Participants were asked if they had taken a prescription drug (not including prescription dietary supplements) in the past 30 days. For participants under age 16, a parent or other proxy provided the information. Those who answered "yes" were asked to show the interviewer the medication containers of all prescription drugs. For each drug reported, the interviewer recorded the product's complete name from the container, if available.

Therapeutic Drug Class (Type of Drugs)

Prescription drugs were classified based on the three- level nested therapeutic classification scheme in Lexicon Plus, a proprietary drug database of Cerner Multum, Inc. [10]. Up to four classes were assigned to each drug. The most commonly cited second level of drug categorical codes were used in this analysis. A drug's therapeutic class does not always align one-to-one with its primary indication. For example, drugs that are used to treat high blood pressure span multiple therapeutic classes (i.e., ACE inhibitors, beta-blockers, diuretics, and calcium channel blockers), and drugs in a single therapeutic class may be used to treat multiple health conditions (e.g., beta-blockers also can be used to treat certain heart diseases). Different approaches to classifying prescription drugs may result in differences in the most commonly used drug types for a given age group.

DATA SOURCE AND METHODS

Data for this chapter are from the National Health and Nutrition Examination Survey (NHANES), a cross-sectional survey conducted by the National Center for Health Statistics and designed to monitor the health and nutritional status of the civilian noninstitutionalized U.S. population. It consists of home interviews followed by standardized physical examinations in mobile examination centers.

The NHANES sample is selected through a complex, multistage probability design. For survey period 2015–2016, non-Hispanic black, non-Hispanic Asian, and Hispanic persons were oversampled; for more information, visit the NHANES website [11]. Non-Hispanic race categories reflect persons reporting only one race; non-Hispanic persons reporting more than one race are included in the total but are not reported separately.

Interview weights were used to account for the differential probabilities of selection, nonresponse, and noncoverage. Taylor series linearization was used to compute variance estimates. Estimates for the population of all ages were age adjusted using the direct method to the projected 2000 U.S. census population using age groups 0–11, 12–19, 20–59, and 60 and over. Pairwise differences between groups were tested using a univariate t statistic. Tests for linear trends by age and over time were evaluated using orthogonal polynomials. The significance level for statistical testing was set at $p < 0.05$. All differences reported are statistically significant unless otherwise indicated. Data management and statistical analyses were conducted using SAS System for Windows version 9.4 (SAS Institute, Inc., Cary, N.C.), SUDAAN version 11.0 (RTI

International, Research Triangle Park, N.C.), and R version 3.5.2 (R Foundation for Statistical Computing).

REFERENCES

[1] Kantor, ED; Rehm, CD; Haas, JS; Chan, AT; Giovannucci, EL. Trends in prescription drug use among adults in the United States from 1999–2012. *JAMA*, 314(17), 1818–31. 2015.

[2] Stone, NJ; Robinson, JG; Lichtenstein, AH; Bairey Merz, CN; Blum, CB; Eckel, RH; et al. 2013 ACC/AHA guideline on the treatment of blood cholesterol to reduce atherosclerotic cardiovascular risk in adults: A report of the American College of Cardiology/American Heart Association Task Force on Practice Guidelines. *J Am Coll Cardiol*, 63(25 Pt B), 2889–934, 2014.

[3] Hales, CM; Kit, BK; Gu, Q; Ogden, CL. Trends in prescription medication use among children and adolescents—United States, 1999–2014. *JAMA*, 319(19), 2009–20, 2018.

[4] Gu, Q; Dillon, CF; Burt, VL. Prescription drug use continues to increase: U.S. prescription drug data for 2007–2008. *NCHS Data Brief*, no 42. Hyattsville, MD: National Center for Heatlh Statistics., 2010.

[5] Akinbami, LJ; Simon, AE; Rossen, LM. Changing trends in asthma prevalence among children. *Pediatrics*, 137(1), 2016.

[6] Xu, G; Strathearn, L; Liu, B; Yang, B; Bao, W. Twenty-year trends in diagnosed attention-deficit/hyperactivity disorder among US children and adolescents, 1997–2016. *JAMA Netw Open*, 1(4), e181471. 2018.

[7] Muntner, P; Carey, RM; Gidding, S; Jones, DW; Taler, SJ; Wright, JT; Whelton, PK. Potential U.S. population impact of the 2017 ACC/AHA High Blood Pressure Guideline. *J Am Coll Cardiol*, 71(2), 109–18. 2018.

[8] Centers for Disease Control and Prevention. *Antibiotic prescribing and use.* Available from: https://www.cdc.gov/antibiotic-use/.

[9] Frenk, SM; Kit, BK; Lukacs, SL; Hicks, LA; Gu, Q. Trends in the use of prescription antibiotics: NHANES 1999–2012. *J Antimicrob Chemother*, 71(1), 251–6, 2016.

[10] National Center for Health Statistics. *National Health and Nutrition Examination Survey 1988–2016 data documentation, codebook, and frequencies: Prescription medications–drug information (RXQ_DRUG).* 2019. Available from: https://wwwn.cdc.gov/ Nchs/ Nhanes/1999-2000/RXQ_DRUG.htm.

[11] National Center for Health Statistics. *NHANES questionnaires, datasets, and related documentation.* 2019. Available from: https://wwwn.cdc.gov/nchs/nhanes/Default.aspx.

In: Prescription Drugs
Editor: Karen Sue McKinney
ISBN: 978-1-53617-288-1

Chapter 5

Prescription Drug Use Among Adults Aged 40–79 in the United States and Canada*

Craig M. Hales, MD, MPH, Jennifer Servais, BSc, Crescent B. Martin, MPH, MA and Dafna Kohen, PhD, MSc

Introduction

Patterns of prescription drug use may reflect underlying patterns of health conditions and health care access in the population. Polypharmacy, often defined as the simultaneous use of five or more prescription drugs, is more common in an aging population where multiple coexisting chronic conditions often occur; however, safety concerns may arise [1]. The United States and Canada share many cultural and historical ties, but with different models for health care delivery [2]. This chapter describes the use of one or

* This is an edited, reformatted and augmented version of NCHS Data Brief, No. 347, dated August 2019.

more and five or more prescription drugs among adults aged 40–79 in the United States and Canada.

Keywords: medication, polypharmacy, National Health and Nutrition Examination Survey (NHANES), Canadian Health Measures Survey (CHMS)

KEY FINDINGS

Data from the National Health and Nutrition Examination Survey and the Canadian Health Measures Survey

- Nearly 7 in 10 adults aged 40–79 used at least 1 prescription drug in the past 30 days in the United States (69.0%) and Canada (65.5%), and around 1 in 5 used at least 5 prescription drugs (22.4% in the United States and 18.8% in Canada).
- Among adults aged 40–59, the most commonly used drug types in the United States were antidepressants, lipid-lowering drugs, and ACE inhibitors; in Canada, they were analgesics, antidepressants, and lipid- lowering drugs.
- Among adults aged 60–79, the most commonly used drug types in the United States were lipid-lowering drugs, antidiabetic agents, and beta blockers; in Canada, they were lipid-lowering drugs, analgesics, and proton pump inhibitors.

WHAT PERCENTAGE OF ADULTS AGED 40–79 IN THE UNITED STATES AND CANADA USED ONE OR MORE AND FIVE OR MORE PRESCRIPTION DRUGS IN THE PAST 30 DAYS?

Among U.S. adults aged 40–79, 69.0% used one or more prescription drugs in the past 30 days and 22.4% used five or more (Figure 1).

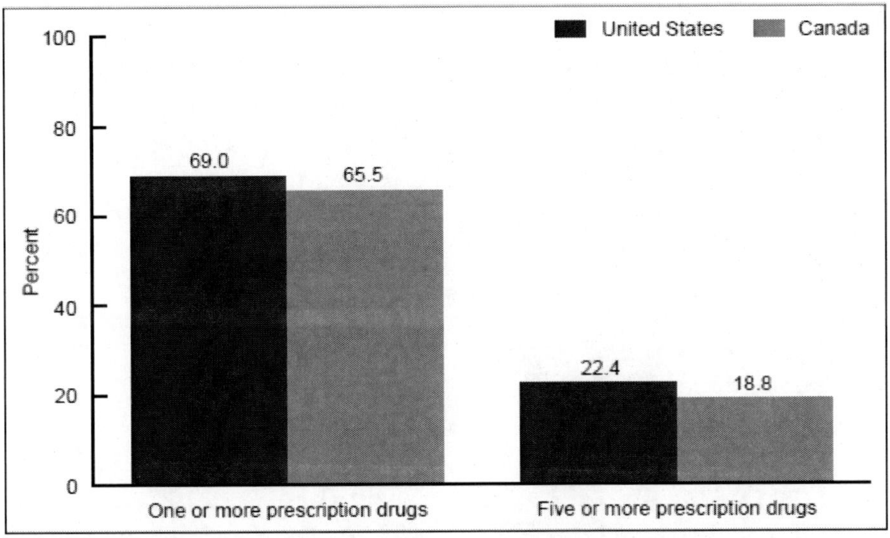

Note: Access data table for Figure 1 at:
https://www.cdc.gov/nchs/data/databriefs/db347_tables-508.pdf#1.
Sources: NCHS, National Health and Nutrition Examination Survey, 2015–2016, and Statistics Canada, Canadian Health Measures Survey, 2016–2017.

Figure 1. Use of one or more and five or more prescription drugs in the past 30 days among adults aged 40–79: United States, 2015–2016, and Canada, 2016–2017.

Among Canadian adults aged 40–79, 65.5% used one or more prescription drugs in the past 30 days and 18.8% used five or more. Use of one or more and five or more prescription drugs was similar between the United States and Canada.

DID USE OF PRESCRIPTION DRUGS IN THE PAST 30 DAYS DIFFER BY SEX AMONG ADULTS IN THE UNITED STATES AND CANADA?

Use of one or more prescription drugs in the past 30 days was greater among women compared with men in both the United States (72.4% compared with 65.2%) and Canada (69.3% compared with 61.7%). Use of five or more prescription drugs was similar between women and men in both the United States (23.5% and 21.1%, respectively) and Canada (19.5% and 18.1%, respectively) (Figure 2). Use of one or more and five or more prescription drugs was similar between the United States and Canada among both men and women.

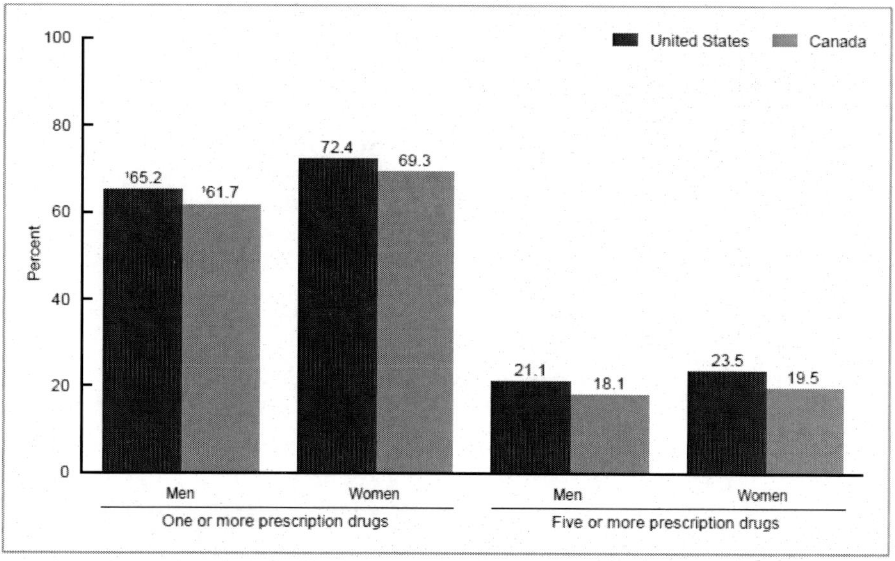

[1]Men significantly different from women.

note: Access data table for Figure 2 at: https://www.cdc.gov/nchs/data/databriefs/db347_tables-508.pdf#2.

sources: NCHS, National Health and Nutrition Examination Survey, 2015–2016, and Statistics Canada, Canadian Health Measures Survey, 2016–2017.

Figure 2. Use of one or more and five or more prescription drugs in the past 30 days among adults aged 40–79, by sex: United States, 2015–2016, and Canada, 2016–2017.

Did Use of Prescription Drugs in the Past 30 Days Differ by Age among Adults in the United States and Canada?

Use of one or more prescription drugs was more common among adults aged 60–79 compared with those aged 40–59 in both the United States (83.6% compared with 59.5%) and Canada (83.3% compared with

53.3%) (Figure 3). Use of five or more prescription drugs was also more common among adults aged 60–79 compared with those aged 40–59 in both the United States (34.5% versus 14.5%) and Canada (30.9% versus 10.4%). Use of one or more and five or more prescription drugs was similar between the United States and Canada among adults aged 40–59 and 60–79.

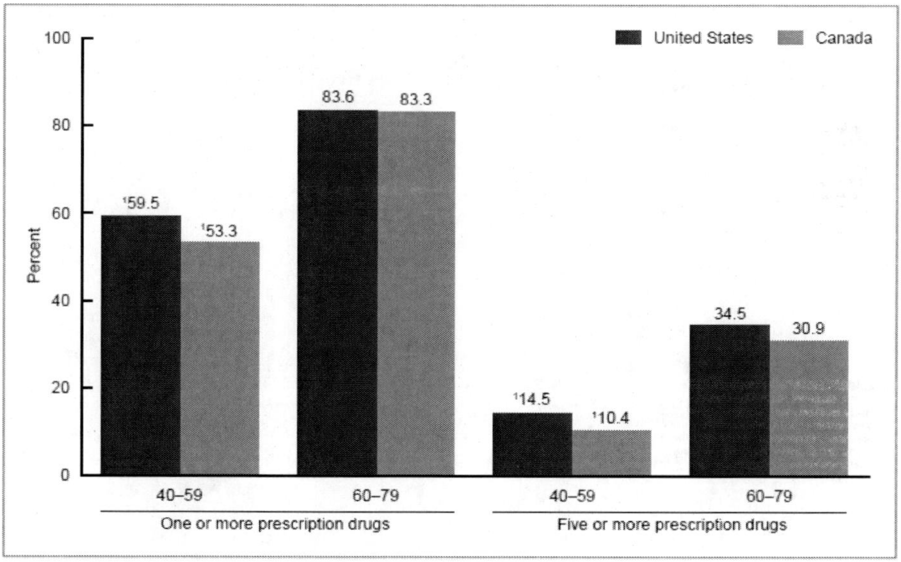

[1]Significantly different from adults aged 60–79.

Note: Access data table for Figure 3 at:
https://www.cdc.gov/nchs/data/databriefs/db347_tables-508.pdf#3.

Sources: NCHS, National Health and Nutrition Examination Survey, 2015–2016, and Statistics Canada, Canadian Health Measures Survey, 2016–2017.

Figure 3. Use of one or more and five or more prescription drugs in the past 30 days among adults aged 40–79, by age group: United States, 2015–2016, and Canada, 2016–2017.

WHAT WERE THE MOST COMMONLY USED TYPES OF PRESCRIPTION DRUGS AMONG ADULTS IN THE UNITED STATES AND CANADA BY AGE?

The top five most common types of prescription drugs used by U.S. and Canadian adults aged 40–79 varied by age and country (Figure 4).

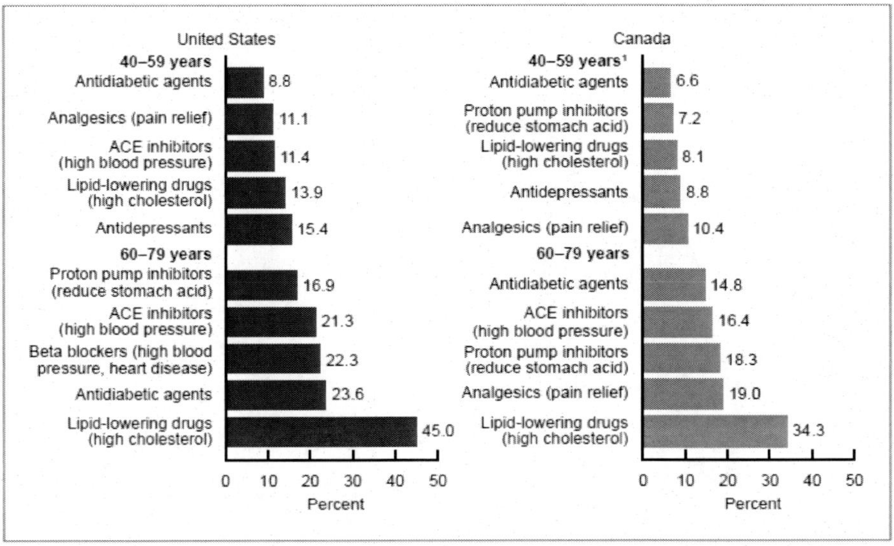

[1]Estimates for Canadian adults aged 40–59 may be unreliable and should be used with caution.

Notes: Primary indication for the use of the drug class is in parentheses. ACE is angiotensin converting enzyme. Access data table for Figure 4 at: https://www.cdc.gov/nchs/data/databriefs/db347_tables-508.pdf#4.

Sources: NCHS, National Health and Nutrition Examination Survey, 2015–2016, and Statistics Canada, Canadian Health Measures Survey, 2016–2017.

Figure 4. Use in the past 30 days of the most common prescription drug types among adults aged 40–79, by age group: United States, 2015–2016, and Canada, 2016–2017.

Among U.S. adults aged 40–59, the most commonly used types of prescription drugs in the past 30 days were antidepressants (15.4%), lipid-lowering drugs (for high cholesterol, 13.9%), angiotensin converting enzyme (ACE) inhibitors (for high blood pressure, 11.4%), analgesics (for pain relief, 11.1%), and antidiabetic agents (8.8%). The most commonly used types of prescription drugs used by Canadian adults aged 40–59 were analgesics (10.4%), antidepressants (8.8%), lipid-lowering drugs (8.1%), proton pump inhibitors (for reducing stomach acid, 7.2%), and antidiabetic agents (6.6%).

Among U.S. adults aged 60–79, the most commonly used types of prescription drugs were lipid-lowering drugs (45.0%), antidiabetic agents (23.6%), beta blockers (for high blood pressure or heart disease, 22.3%), ACE inhibitors (21.3%), and proton pump inhibitors (16.9%). The most commonly used types of prescription drugs among Canadian adults aged 60–79 were lipid-lowering drugs (34.3%), analgesics (19.0%), proton pump inhibitors (18.3%), ACE inhibitors (16.4%), and antidiabetic agents (14.8%).

CONCLUSION

Use of prescription drugs was similar in the United States and Canada. Nearly 7 in 10 adults aged 40–79 used at least 1 prescription drug in the past 30 days, and around 1 in 5 used at least 5 prescription drugs. In both the United States and Canada, use of one or more prescription drugs was higher among women compared with men, but use of five or more prescription drugs was similar among women and men. In both the United States and Canada, use of one or more and five or more prescription drugs was more common among adults aged 60–79 compared with adults aged 40–59.

The top five most common types of prescription drugs used by U.S. and Canadian adults varied by age and country. Among adults aged 40–59, antidepressants were the most commonly used drug type among U.S. adults, while analgesics were the most commonly used drug type by Canadian adults. Among both U.S. and Canadian adults aged 60–79, lipid-lowering drugs were the most common type of drug used. The second most common drug type among U.S. adults aged 60–79 was antidiabetic agents, whereas antidiabetic agents were the fifth-most common drug type used by

Canadian adults aged 60–79. Analgesics (for pain relief) was the second most common drug type among Canadian adults aged 60–79, whereas analgesics did not rank in the top five most commonly used drug types among U.S. adults aged 60–79.

Monitoring the use of prescription drugs provides insights into the health and health care of U.S. and Canadian adults. The age distribution of the U.S. and Canadian populations is similar, with adults aged 40–79 making up 44% of the population in the United States and 48% in Canada in 2016 [3, 4]. The use of one or more and five or more medications among adults aged 40–79 is similar between the United States and Canada, despite substantial differences in their health care systems. However, patterns of the most commonly used drug types are different in the two countries.

DEFINITIONS

Prescription Drug Use

National Health and Nutrition Examination Survey (NHANES) participants were asked if they had taken a prescription drug in the past 30 days. In the Canadian Health Measures Survey (CHMS), participants were asked if they had taken or used any medications that have been prescribed or administered by a health professional in the past month. In both surveys, those who answered "yes" were asked to show the interviewer the medication containers of all prescription drugs. For each drug reported, the interviewer recorded the product's complete name from the container, if available.

Drug Type

In NHANES, prescription drugs were classified based on the second level of therapeutic classification scheme in the Multum Lexicon Plus drug database [5]. In CHMS, prescription drugs were coded using the

Anatomical Therapeutic Chemical (ATC) classification system developed by the World Health Organization [6]. For this analysis, ATC codes were also categorized based on the second level of therapeutic classification scheme in the Multum Lexicon Plus drug database for comparability with NHANES.

A drug's therapeutic class does not always align one-to-one with its primary indication. For example, drugs that are used to treat high blood pressure span multiple therapeutic classes (i.e., ACE inhibitors, beta blockers, diuretics, and calcium channel blockers) and drugs in a single therapeutic class may be used to treat multiple health conditions (e.g., beta blockers also can be used to treat certain heart diseases). Different approaches to drug classification schemes may result in differences in the most commonly used drugs for a given group.

DATA SOURCES AND METHODS

Data for this chapter are from NHANES and CHMS. NHANES and CHMS are cross-sectional surveys designed to provide nationally representative estimates of the noninstitutionalized populations of the United States and Canada, respectively. NHANES is conducted by the National Center for Health Statistics and CHMS is conducted by Statistics Canada. The surveys consist of home interviews followed by standardized physical examinations in mobile examination centers.

The samples for both surveys are selected through a complex, multistage probability design, and sample weights—which account for the differential probabilities of selection, nonresponse, and noncoverage—are incorporated into the estimation process. Standard errors for CHMS were estimated using the bootstrap method; estimates with a high coefficient of variation between 16.6 and 33.3 may be unreliable and were flagged as "use with caution." For NHANES, standard errors were estimated by Taylor series linearization. Both the bootstrap and Taylor series linearization methods account for the design features of the survey. Differences in the prevalence of prescription drug use between men and women, adults aged 40–59 and 60–79, and between Canada and the United States were tested using a univariate *t* statistic with an α level of 0.05. All differences reported are statistically significant unless otherwise indicated. Data management and statistical analyses were conducted using SAS System for Windows versions 9.3 and 9.4 (SAS Institute, Inc., Cary, N.C.), SUDAAN version 11.0 (RTI International, Research Triangle Park, N.C.), and R version 3.5.2 (R Foundation for Statistical Computing, Vienna, Austria), including the R survey package [7] to account for the complex sample design.

References

[1] Wastesson JW, Morin L, Tan ECK, Johnell K. An update on the clinical consequences of polypharmacy in older adults: A narrative review. *Expert Opin Drug Saf* 17(12):1185–96. 2018.

[2] Sanmartin C, Berthelot JM, Ng E, Murphy K, Blackwell DL, Gentleman JF, et al. Comparing health and health care use in Canada and the United States. *Health Aff* (Millwood) 25(4):1133–42. 2006. Available from: https://doi.org/10.1377/hlthaff.25.4.1133.

[3] U.S. Census Bureau. American Fact Finder. Available from: https://factfinder.census.gov/faces/nav/jsf/pages/index.xhtml.

[4] Statistics Canada. *Census Program.* Available from: https://www12.statcan.gc.ca/census- recensement/index-eng.cfm.

[5] National Center for Health Statistics. *NHANES 1988–2016 data documentation, codebook, and frequencies: Prescription medications - drug information (RXQ_DRUG).* Available from: https://wwwn.cdc.gov/Nchs/Nhanes/1999-2000/RXQ_DRUG.htm.

[6] WHO Collaborating Centre for Drug Statistics Methodology. *International language for drug utilization research.* 2019. Available from: https://www.whocc.no/.

[7] Lumley T. Survey: *Analysis of complex survey samples.* R package version 3.35. 2018.

In: Prescription Drugs
Editor: Karen Sue McKinney
ISBN: 978-1-53617-288-1

Chapter 6

TO AMEND TITLE XVIII OF THE SOCIAL SECURITY ACT TO REQUIRE PRESCRIPTION DRUG PLAN SPONSORS UNDER THE MEDICARE PROGRAM TO ESTABLISH DRUG MANAGEMENT PROGRAMS FOR AT-RISK BENEFICIARIES*

Committee on Energy and Commerce

Mr. Walden, from the Committee on Energy and Commerce, submitted the following report [To accompany H.R. 5675]

[Including cost estimate of the Congressional Budget Office]

The Committee on Energy and Commerce, to whom was referred the bill (H.R. 5675) to amend title XVIII of the Social Security Act to require prescription drug plan sponsors under the Medicare program to establish drug management programs for at-risk beneficiaries, having considered the

---

* This is an edited, reformatted and augmented version of Committed to the Committee of the Whole House on the State of the Union, One Hundred Fifteenth Congress, 2nd Session, dated June 12, 2018.

same, report favorably thereon without amendment and recommend that the bill do pass.

PURPOSE AND SUMMARY

H.R. 5675 was introduced on May 3, 2018, by Rep. Gus Bilirakis (R–FL), Rep. Ben Ray Luja´ n (D–NM), Rep. Peter Roskam (R–IL), and Rep. Sander Levin (D–MI) to build off of work done in the Comprehensive Addiction Recovery Act (CARA), and will require prescription drug plan sponsors under the Medicare program to establish drug management programs for at-risk beneficiaries.

BACKGROUND AND NEED FOR LEGISLATION

The Medicare program serves as the healthcare coverage provider to over 58 million beneficiaries. This number is projected to rise to over 80 million by 2030. In serving the over age 65 population, Medicare accounts for a large share of total opioid prescriptions. In 2016, one out of every three beneficiaries was prescribed an opioid through Medicare Part D. In total, this equates to almost 80 million prescriptions and $4 billion in Medicare Part D spending. While many Medicare beneficiaries with serious pain-related conditions are being properly prescribed opioids, there is mounting evidence of opioid misuse in the Medicare system. As more seniors and individuals with disabilities come into the program, the challenges of fraud, misuse, and abuse will only increase.

This bill seeks to accelerate the development and use of drug management programs for at-risk beneficiaries within the Medicare program by requiring all Medicare prescription drug plans to establish these programs. Under current law, prescription drug plan sponsors are authorized to create drug management programs, but are not required to do so.

COMMITTEE ACTION

On April 11 and 12, 2018, the Subcommittee on Health held a hearing entitled "Combating the Opioid Crisis: Improving the Ability of Medicare and Medicaid to Provide Care for Patients" to review legislation related to the opioid epidemic. The Subcommittee received testimony from:

- Kimberly Brandt, Principal Deputy Administrator for Operations, Centers for Medicare and Medicaid Services, U.S. Department of Health and Human Services;
- Michael Botticelli, Executive Director, Grayken Center for Addiction, Boston Medical Center;
- Toby Douglas, Senior Vice President, Medicaid Solutions, Centene Corporation;
- David Guth, CEO, Centerstone;
- John Kravitz, CIO, Geisinger Health System; and,
- Sam Srivastava, CEO, Magellan Health.

On April 25, 2018, the Subcommittee on Health met in open markup session and forwarded a discussion draft, entitled "Mandatory Lock-In," without amendment, to the full Committee by a voice vote. On May 9, 2018, the full Committee on Energy and Commerce met in open markup session and ordered H.R. 5675, without amendment, favorable reported to the House by a voice vote. H.R. 5675 was similar to the discussion draft forwarded by the Subcommittee.

COMMITTEE VOTES

Clause 3(b) of rule XIII requires the Committee to list the record votes on the motion to report legislation and amendments thereto. There were no record votes taken in connection with ordering H.R. 5675 reported.

OVERSIGHT FINDINGS AND RECOMMENDATIONS

Pursuant to clause 2(b)(1) of rule X and clause 3(c)(1) of rule XIII, the Committee held a hearing and made findings that are reflected in this chapter.

NEW BUDGET AUTHORITY, ENTITLEMENT AUTHORITY, AND TAX EXPENDITURES

Pursuant to clause 3(c)(2) of rule XIII, the Committee finds that H.R. 5675 would result in no new or increased budget authority, entitlement authority, or tax expenditures or revenues.

CONGRESSIONAL BUDGET OFFICE ESTIMATE

Pursuant to clause 3(c)(3) of rule XIII, the following is the cost estimate provided by the Congressional Budget Office pursuant to section 402 of the Congressional Budget Act of 1974:

U.S. Congress, Congressional Budget Office,
Washington, DC, June 6, 2018.

Hon. Greg Walden,
Chairman, Committee on Energy and Commerce,
House of Representatives, Washington, DC.

Dear Mr. Chairman: The Congressional Budget Office has prepared the enclosed document with cost estimates for the opioid-related legislation ordered to be reported on May 9 and May 17, 2018.

If you wish further details on this estimate, we will be pleased to provide them. The CBO staff contacts are Tom Bradley and Chad Chirico.

Sincerely,

Mark P. Hadley
(For Keith Hall, Director).

Opioid Legislation

Summary: On May 9 and May 17, 2018, the House Committee on Energy and Commerce ordered 59 bills to be reported related to the nation's response to the opioid epidemic. Generally, the bills would:

- Provide grants to facilities and providers that treat people with substance use disorders,
- Direct various agencies within the Department of Health and Human Services (HHS) to explore nonopioid approaches to treating pain and to educate providers about those alternatives,
- Modify requirements under Medicaid and Medicare for prescribing controlled substances,
- Expand Medicaid coverage for substance abuse treatment, and
- Direct the Food and Drug Administration (FDA) to modify its oversight of opioid drugs and other medications that are used to manage pain.

Because of the large number of related bills ordered reported by the Committee, CBO is publishing a single comprehensive document that includes estimates for each piece of legislation.

CBO estimates that enacting 20 of the bills would affect direct spending, and 2 of the bills would affect revenues; therefore, pay-as-you-go procedures apply for those bills.

CBO estimates that enacting H.R. 4998, the Health Insurance for Former Foster Youth Act, would increase net direct spending by more than $2.5 billion and on-budget deficits by more than $5 billion in at least one of the four consecutive 10-year periods beginning in 2029. None of the remaining 58 bills included in this estimate would increase net direct spending by more than $2.5 billion or on-budget deficits by more than $5 billion in any of the four consecutive 10-year periods beginning in 2029.

One of the bills reviewed for this document, H.R. 5795, would impose both intergovernmental and private-sector mandates as defined in the Unfunded Mandates Reform Act (UMRA). CBO estimates that the costs of those mandates on public and private entities would fall below the thresholds in UMRA ($80 million and $160 million, respectively, in 2018, adjusted annually for inflation). Five bills, H.R. 5228, H.R. 5333, H.R. 5554, H.R. 5687, and H.R. 5811, would impose private-sector mandates as defined in UMRA. CBO estimates that the costs of the mandates in three of the bills (H.R. 5333, H.R. 5554, and H.R. 5811) would not exceed the UMRA threshold for private entities. Because CBO is uncertain how federal agencies would implement new authority granted in the other two bills, H.R. 5228 and H.R. 5687, CBO cannot determine whether the costs of those mandates would exceed the UMRA threshold.

Estimated cost to the Federal Government: The estimates in this document do not include the effects of interactions among the bills. If all 59 bills were combined and enacted as one piece of legislation, the budgetary effects would be different from the sum of the estimates in this document, although CBO expects that any such differences would be small. The costs of this legislation fall within budget functions 550 (health), 570 (Medicare), 750 (administration of justice), and 800 (general government).

Basis of estimate: For this estimate, CBO assumes that all of the legislation will be enacted late in 2018 and that authorized and estimated amounts will be appropriated each year. Outlays for discretionary programs are estimated based on historical spending patterns for similar programs.

Uncertainty

CBO aims to produce estimates that generally reflect the middle of a range of the most likely budgetary outcomes that would result if the legislation was enacted. Because data on the utilization of mental health and substance abuse treatment under Medicaid and Medicare is scarce, CBO cannot precisely predict how patients or providers would respond to some policy changes or what budgetary effects would result. In addition, several of the bills would give the Department of Health and Human Services (HHS) considerable latitude in designing and implementing policies. Budgetary effects could differ from those provided in CBO's analyses depending on those decisions.

Direct Spending and Revenues

Table 1 lists the 22 bills of the 59 ordered to be reported that would affect direct spending or revenues.

Legislation Primarily Affecting Medicaid. The following nine bills would affect direct spending for the Medicaid program.

H.R. 1925, the At-Risk Youth Medicaid Protection Act of 2017, would require states to suspend, rather than terminate, Medicaid eligibility for juvenile enrollees (generally under 21 years of age) who become inmates of public correctional institutions. States also would have to redetermine those enrollees' Medicaid eligibility before their release and restore their coverage upon release if they qualify for the program. States would be required to process Medicaid applications submitted by or on behalf of juveniles in public correctional institutions who were not enrolled in Medicaid before becoming inmates and ensure that Medicaid coverage is provided when they are released if they are found to be eligible.

On the basis of an analysis of juvenile incarceration trends and of the per enrollee spending for Medicaid foster care children, who have a similar health profile to incarcerated juveniles, CBO estimates that implementing the bill would cost $75 million over the 2019–2028 period.

H.R. 4998, the Health Insurance for Former Foster Youth Act, would require states to provide Medicaid coverage to adults up to age 25 who had aged out of foster care in any state. Under current law, such coverage is mandatory only if the former foster care youth has aged out in the state in which the individual applies for coverage. The policy also would apply to former foster children who had been in foster care upon turning 14 years of age but subsequently left foster care to enter into a legal guardianship with a kinship caregiver. The provisions would take effect respect for foster youth who turn 18 on or after January 1, 2023. On the basis of spending for Medicaid foster care children and data from the Census Bureau regarding annual migration rates between states, CBO estimates that implementing the bill would cost $171 million over the 2019–2028 period.

H.R. 5477, the Rural Development of Opioid Capacity Services Act, would direct the Secretary of HHS to conduct a five-year demonstration to increase the number and ability of providers participating in Medicaid to provide treatment for substance use disorders. On the basis of an analysis of federal and state spending for treatment of substance use disorders and the prevalence of such disorders, CBO estimates that enacting the bill would increase direct spending by $301 million over the 2019–2028 period.

H.R. 5583, a bill to amend title XI of the Social Security Act to require States to annually report on certain adult health quality measures, and for other purposes, would require states to include behavioral health indicators in their annual reports on the quality of care under Medicaid. Although the bill would add a requirement for states, CBO estimates that its enactment would not have a significant budgetary effect because most states have systems in place for reporting such measures to the federal government.

Table 1. Estimated Changes in Mandatory Spending and Revenues

	By fiscal year, in millions of dollars—												
	2018	2019	2020	2021	2022	2023	2024	2025	2026	2027	2028	2019-2023	2019-2028
INCREASES OR DECREASES (–) IN DIRECT SPENDING													
Legislation Primarily Affecting Medicaid:													
H.R. 1925, At-Risk Youth Medicaid Protection Act of 2017	0	*	5	5	5	10	10	10	10	10	10	25	75
H.R. 4998, Health Insurance for Former Foster Youth Act	0	0	0	0	0	*	10	21	33	46	61	*	171
H.R. 5477, Rural Development of Opioid Capacity Services Act	0	13	35	58	68	83	27	9	3	3	3	256	301
H.R. 5583, a bill to amend title XI of the Social Security Act to require States to annually report on certain adult health quality measures,and for other purposes	0	*	*	*	*	*	*	*	*	*	*	*	*
H.R. 5797, IMD CARE Act	0	38	158	251	265	279	0	0	0	0	0	991	991
H.R. 5799, Medicaid DRUG Improvement Act[a]	0	*	*	1	1	1	1	1	1	1	1	2	5
H.R. 5801 Medicaid Providers Are Required To Note Experiences in Record Systems to Help In-Need Patients (PARTNERSHIP) Act[a]	0	*	*	*	*	*	*	*	*	*	*	*	*
H.R. 5808, Medicaid Pharmaceutical Home Act of 2018[a]	0	– 2	– 1	– 1	– 1	– 1	– 2	– 2	– 2	– 2	– 2	– 4	– 13
H.R. 5810, Medicaid Health HOME Act	0	94	58	62	56	52	48	43	38	32	25	323	509
Legislation Primarily Affecting Medicare:													
H.R. 3528, Every Prescription Conveyed Securely Act	0	0	0	– 24	– 35	– 33	– 30	– 33	– 32	– 31	– 32	– 92	– 250
H.R. 4841, Standardizing Electronic Prior Authorization for Safe Prescribing Act of 2018	0	0	0	*	*	*	*	*	*	*	*	*	*
H.R. 5603, Access to Telehealth Services for Opioid Use Disorders Act	0	2	*	*	*	1	1	1	2	2	2	3	11
H.R. 5605, Advancing High Quality Treatment for Opioid Use Disorders in Medicare Act	0	0	0	15	26	24	23	23	10	1	*	65	122

Table 1. (Continued)

	By fiscal year, in millions of dollars—												
	2018	2019	2020	2021	2022	2023	2024	2025	2026	2027	2028	2019-2023	2019-2028
H.R. 5675, a bill to amend title XVIII of the Social Security Act to require prescription drug plan sponsors under the Medicare program to establish drug management programs for at-risk beneficiaries ...	0	0	0	– 6	– 7	– 7	– 7	– 8	– 9	– 9	– 11	– 20	– 64
H.R. 5684, Protecting Seniors From Opioid Abuse Act	0	0	0	*	*	*	*	*	*	*	*	*	* H.R.
5796, Responsible Education Achieves Care and Healthy Out-comes for Users' Treatment Act of 2018	0	10	25	50	10	5	0	0	0	0	0	100	100
H.R. 5798, Opioid Screening and Chronic Pain Management Alter-natives for Seniors Act	0	0	*	1	1	1	1	1	1	1	1	2	5
H.R. 5804, Post-Surgical Injections as an Opioid Alternative Act[a]	0	0	25	30	25	20	10	5	0	0	0	100	115
H.R. 5809, Postoperative Opioid Prevention Act of 2018	0	0	0	0	10	15	20	25	30	35	45	25	180
Legislation Primarily Affecting the Food and Drug Administration:													
H.R. 5333, Over-the-Counter Monograph Safety, Innovation, and Reform Act of 2018[a]	0	0	*	*	*	*	*	*	*	*	*	*	*
INCREASES OR DECREASES (–) IN REVENUES[b]													
H.R. 5752, Stop Illicit Drug Importation Act of 2018	0	*	*	*	*	*	*	*	*	*	*	*	*

Annual amounts may not sum to totals because of rounding. * = between ¥$500,000 and $500,000. Budget authority is equivalent to outlays.

[a] This bill also would affect spending subject to appropriation.

[b] One additional bill, H.R. 5228, the Stop Counterfeit Drugs by Regulating and Enhancing Enforcement Now Act, would have a negligible effect on revenues.

H.R. 5797, the IMD CARE Act, would expand Medicaid coverage for people with opioid use disorder who are in institutions for mental disease (IMDs) for up to 30 days per year. Under a current-law policy known as the IMD exclusion, the federal government generally does not make matching payments to state Medicaid programs for most services provided by IMDs to adults between the ages of 21 and 64. Recent administrative changes have made federal financing for IMDs available in limited circumstances, but the statutory prohibition remains in place. CBO analyzed several data sets, primarily those collected by the Substance Abuse and Mental Health Services Administration (SAMHSA), to estimate current federal spending under Medicaid for IMD services and to estimate spending under H.R. 5797. Using that analysis, CBO estimates that enacting H.R. 5797 would increase direct spending by $991 million over the 2019–2028 period.

H.R. 5799, the Medicaid DRUG Improvement Act, would require state Medicaid programs to implement additional reviews of opioid prescriptions, monitor concurrent prescribing of opioids and certain other drugs, and monitor use of antipsychotic drugs by children. CBO estimates that the bill would increase direct spending by $5 million over the 2019–2028 period to cover the administrative costs of complying with those requirements. On the basis of stakeholder feedback, CBO expects that the bill would not have a significant effect on Medicaid spending for prescription drugs because many of the bill's requirements would duplicate current efforts to curb opioid and antipsychotic drug use. (If enacted, H.R. 5799 also would affect spending subject to appropriation; CBO has not completed an estimate of that amount.)

H.R. 5801, the Medicaid Providers Are Required To Note Experiences in Record Systems to Help In-Need Patients (PARTNERSHIP) Act, would require providers who are permitted to prescribe controlled substances and who participate in Medicaid to query prescription drug monitoring programs (PDMPs) before prescribing controlled substances to Medicaid patients. PDMPs are statewide electronic databases that collect data on controlled substances dispensed in the state. The bill also would require PDMPs to comply with certain data and system criteria, and it would provide additional federal matching funds to certain states to help cover administrative costs. On the basis of a literature review and stakeholder feedback, CBO estimates that the net budgetary effect of enacting H.R. 5801 would be insignificant. Costs for states to come into compliance with the systems and administrative requirements would be roughly offset by savings from small reductions in the number of controlled substances paid for by Medicaid under the proposal. (If enacted, H.R. 5801 also would affect spending subject to appropriation; CBO has not completed an estimate of that amount.)

H.R. 5808, the Medicaid Pharmaceutical Home Act of 2018, would require state Medicaid programs to operate pharmacy programs that would identify people at high risk of abusing controlled substances and require those patients to use a limited number of providers and pharmacies. Although nearly all state Medicaid programs currently meet such a requirement, a small number of high-risk Medicaid beneficiaries are not now monitored. Based on an analysis of information about similar state and federal programs, CBO estimates that net Medicaid spending under the bill would decrease by $13 million over the 2019–2028 period. That amount represents a small increase in administrative costs and a small reduction in the number of controlled substances paid for by Medicaid under the proposal. (If enacted, H.R. 5808 also would affect spending subject to appropriation; CBO has not completed an estimate of that amount.)

H.R. 5810, the Medicaid Health HOME Act, would allow states to receive six months of enhanced federal Medicaid funding for programs that coordinate care for people with substance use disorders. Based on enrollment and spending data from states that currently participate in Medicaid's Health Homes program, CBO estimates that the expansion would cost approximately $469 million over the 2019–2028 period. The bill also would require states to cover all FDA-approved drugs used in medication-assisted treatment for five years, although states could seek a waiver from that requirement. (Medication-assisted treatment combines behavioral therapy and pharmaceutical treatment for substance use disorders.) Under current law, states already cover most FDA-approved drugs used in such programs in some capacity, although a few exclude methadone dispensed by opioid treatment programs. CBO estimates that a small share of those states would begin to cover methadone if this bill was enacted at a federal cost of about $39 million over the 2019–2028 period. In sum, CBO estimates that the enacting H.R. 5810 would increase direct spending by $509 million over the 2019–2028 period.

Legislation Primarily Affecting Medicare. The following ten bills would affect direct spending for the Medicare program.

H.R. 3528, the Every Prescription Conveyed Securely Act, would require prescriptions for controlled substances covered under Medicare Part D to be transmitted electronically, starting on January 1, 2021. Based on CBO's analysis of prescription drug spending, spending for controlled substances is a small share of total drug spending. CBO also assumes a small share of those prescriptions would not be filled because they are not converted to an electronic format. Therefore, CBO expects that enacting H.R. 3528 would reduce the number of prescriptions filled and estimates that Medicare spending would be reduced by $250 million over the 2019–2028 period.

H.R. 4841, the Standardizing Electronic Prior Authorization for Safe Prescribing Act of 2018, would require health care professionals to submit prior authorization requests electronically, starting on January 1, 2021, for drugs covered under Medicare Part D. Taking into account that many prescribers already use electronic methods to submit such requests, CBO estimates that enacting H.R. 4841 would not significantly affect direct spending for Part D.

H.R. 5603, the Access to Telehealth Services for Opioid Use Disorders Act, would permit the Secretary of HHS to lift current geographic and other restrictions on coverage of telehealth services under Medicare for treatment of substance use disorders or co-occurring mental health disorders. Under the bill, the Secretary of HHS would be directed to encourage other payers to coordinate payments for opioid use disorder treatments and to evaluate the extent to which the demonstration reduces hospitalizations, increases the use of medication-assisted treatments, and improves the health outcomes of individuals with opioid use disorders during and after the demonstration. Based on current use of Medicare telehealth services for treatment of substance use disorders, CBO estimates that expanding that coverage would increase direct spending by $11 million over the 2019–2028 period.

H.R. 5605, the Advancing High Quality Treatment for Opioid Use Disorders in Medicare Act, would establish a five-year demonstration program to increase access to treatment for opioid use disorder. The demonstration would provide incentive payments and funding for care management services based on criteria such as patient engagement, use of evidence-based treatments, and treatment length and intensity. Under the bill, the Secretary of HHS would be directed to encourage other payers to coordinate payments for opioid use disorder treatments and to evaluate the extent to which the demonstration reduces hospitalizations, increases the use of medication-assisted treatments, and improves the health outcomes of individuals with opioid use disorders during and after the demonstration. Based on historical utilization of opioid use disorder treatments and projected spending on incentive payments and care management fees, CBO estimates that increased use of treatment services and the demonstration's incentive payments would increase direct spending by $122 million over the 2019–2028 period.

H.R. 5675, a bill to amend title XVIII of the Social Security Act to require prescription drug plan sponsors under the Medicare program to establish drug management programs for at-risk beneficiaries, would require Part D prescription drug plans to provide drug management programs for Medicare beneficiaries who are at risk for prescription drug abuse. (Under current law, Part D plans are permitted but not required to establish such programs as of 2019.) Based on an analysis of the number of plans currently providing those programs, CBO estimates that enacting H.R. 5675 would lower federal spending by $64 million over the 2019–2028 period by reducing the number of prescriptions filled and Medicare's payments for controlled substances.

H.R. 5684, the Protecting Seniors From Opioid Abuse Act, would expand medication therapy management programs under Medicare Part D to include beneficiaries who are at risk for prescription drug abuse.

Because relatively few beneficiaries would be affected by this bill, CBO estimates that its enactment would not significantly affect direct spending for Part D.

H.R. 5796, the Responsible Education Achieves Care and Healthy Outcomes for Users' Treatment Act of 2018, would allow the Secretary of HHS to award grants to certain organizations that provide technical assistance and education to high-volume prescribers of opioids. The bill would appropriate $100 million for fiscal year 2019. Based on historical spending patterns for similar activities, CBO estimates that implementing H.R. 5796 would cost $100 million over the 2019–2028 period.

H.R. 5798, the Opioid Screening and Chronic Pain Management Alternatives for Seniors Act, would add an assessment of current opioid prescriptions and screening for opioid use disorder to the Welcome to Medicare Initial Preventive Physical Examination. Based on historical use of the examinations and pain management alternatives, CBO expects that enacting the bill would increase use of pain management services and estimates that direct spending would increase by $5 million over the 2019–2028 period.

H.R. 5804, the Post-Surgical Injections as an Opioid Alternative Act, would freeze the Medicare payment rate for certain analgesic injections provided in ambulatory surgical centers (ASCs). (For injections identified by specific billing codes, Medicare would pay the 2016 rate, which is higher than the current rate, during the 2020–2024 period.) Based on current utilization in the ASC setting, CBO estimates that enacting the legislation would increase direct spending by about $115 million over the 2019–2028 period. (If enacted, H.R. 5804 also would affect spending subject to appropriation; see Table 3.)

H.R. 5809, the Postoperative Opioid Prevention Act of 2018, would create an additional payment under Medicare for nonopioid analgesics. Under current law, certain new drugs and devices may receive an additional payment—separate from the bundled payment for a surgical procedure—in outpatient hospital departments and ambulatory surgical centers. The bill would allow nonopioid analgesics to qualify for a five-year period of additional payments. Based on its assessment of current spending for analgesics and on the probability of new nonopioid analgesics coming to market, CBO estimates that H.R. 5809 would increase direct spending by about $180 million over the 2019–2028 period.

Legislation Primarily Affecting the Food and Drug Administration. One bill related to the FDA would affect direct spending.

H.R. 5333, the Over-the-Counter Monograph Safety, Innovation, and Reform Act of 2018, would change the way that the FDA regulates the marketing of over-the-counter (OTC) medicines, and it would authorize that agency to grant 18 months of exclusive market protection for certain qualifying OTC drugs, thus delaying the entry of other versions of the same qualifying OTC product. Medicaid currently provides some coverage for OTC medicines, but only if a medicine is the least costly alternative in its drug class. On the basis of stakeholder feedback, CBO expects that delaying the availability of additional OTC versions of a drug would not significantly affect the average net price paid by Medicaid. As a result, CBO estimates that enacting H.R. 5333 would have a negligible effect on the federal budget. (If enacted, H.R. 5333 also would affect spending subject to appropriation; see Table 3.)

Legislation with Revenue Effects. Two bills would affect revenues. However, CBO estimates that one bill, H.R. 5228, the Stop Counterfeit Drugs by Regulating and Enhancing Enforcement Now Act, would have only a negligible effect.

H.R. 5752, the Stop Illicit Drug Importation Act of 2018, would amend the Federal, Food, Drug, and Cosmetic Act (FDCA) to strengthen the FDA's seizure powers and enhance its authority to detain, refuse, seize, or destroy illegal products offered for import. The legislation would subject more people to debarment under the FDCA and thus increase the potential for violations, and subsequently, the assessment of civil penalties, which are recorded in the budget as revenues. CBO estimates that those collections would result in an insignificant increase in revenues. Because H.R. 5752 would prohibit the importation of drugs that are in the process of being scheduled, it also could reduce amounts collected in customs duties. CBO anticipates that the result would be a negligible decrease in revenues. With those results taken together, CBO estimates, enacting H.R.

5752 would generate an insignificant net increase in revenues over the 2019–2028 period.

Spending Subject to Appropriation

For this document, CBO has grouped bills with spending that would be subject to appropriation into four general categories:

- Bills that would have no budgetary effect,
- Bills with provisions that would authorize specified amounts to be appropriated (see Table 2),
- Bills with provisions for which CBO has estimated an authorization of appropriations (see Table 3), and
- Bills with provisions that would affect spending subject to appropriation for which CBO has not yet completed an estimate.

No Budgetary Effect. CBO estimates that 6 of the 59 bills would have no effect on direct spending, revenues, or spending subject to appropriation.

H.R. 3192, the CHIP Mental Health Parity Act, would require all Children's Health Insurance Program (CHIP) plans to cover mental health and substance abuse treatment. In addition, states would not be allowed to impose financial or utilization limits on mental health treatment that are lower than limits placed on physical health treatment. Based on information from the Centers for Medicare and Medicaid Services, CBO estimates that enacting the bill would have no budgetary effect because all CHIP enrollees are already in plans that meet those requirements.

H.R. 3331, a bill to amend title XI of the Social Security Act to promote testing of incentive payments for behavioral health providers for adoption and use of certified electronic health record technology, would give the Center for Medicare and Medicaid Innovation (CMMI) explicit authorization to test a program offering incentive payments to behavioral health providers that adopt and use certified electronic health record technology. Because it is already clear to CMMI that it has that authority, CBO estimates that enacting the legislation would not affect federal spending.

H.R. 5202, the Ensuring Patient Access to Substance Use Disorder Treatments Act of 2018, would clarify permission for pharmacists to deliver controlled substances to providers under certain circumstances. Because this provision would codify current practice, CBO estimates that H.R. 5202 would not affect direct spending or revenues during the 2019–2028 period.

H.R. 5685, the Medicare Opioid Safety Education Act of 2018, would require the Secretary of HHS to include information on opioid use, pain management, and nonopioid pain management treatments in future editions of *Medicare & You,* the program's handbook for beneficiaries, starting on January 1, 2019. Because H.R. 5685 would add information to an existing administrative document, CBO estimates that enacting the bill would have no budgetary effect.

H.R. 5686, the Medicare Clear Health Options in Care for Enrollees Act of 2018, would require prescription drug plans that provide coverage under Medicare Part D to furnish information to beneficiaries about the risks of opioid use and the availability of alternative treatments for pain. CBO estimates that enacting the bill would not affect direct spending because the required activities would not impose significant administrative costs.

H.R. 5716, the Commit to Opioid Medical Prescriber Accountability and Safety for Seniors Act, would require the Secretary of HHS on an annual basis to identify high prescribers of opioids and furnish them with information about proper prescribing methods. Because HHS already has the capacity to meet those requirements, CBO estimates that enacting that provision would not impose additional administrative costs on the agency.

Specified Authorizations. Table 2 lists the ten bills that would authorize specified amounts to be appropriated over the 2019–2023 period. Spending from those authorized amounts would be subject to appropriation.

Table 2. Estimated Spending Subject to Appropriation for Bills with Specified Authorizations

	By fiscal year, in millions of dollars—						
	2018	**2019**	**2020**	**2021**	**2022**	**2023**	**2019-2023**
INCREASES IN SPENDING SUBJECT TO APPROPRIATION							
H.R. 4684, Ensuring Access to Quality Sober Living Act:							
Authorization Level	0	3	0	0	0	0	3
Estimated Outlays	0	1	2	*	*	*	3
H.R. 5102, Substance Use Disorder Workforce Loan Repayment Act of 2018:							
Authorization Level	0	25	25	25	25	25	125
Estimated Outlays	0	9	19	23	25	25	100
H.R. 5176, Preventing Overdoses While in Emergency Rooms Act of 2018:							
Authorization Level	0	50	0	0	0	0	50
Estimated Outlays	0	16	26	6	2	1	50
H.R. 5197, Alternatives to Opioids (ALTO) in the Emergency Department Act:							
Authorization Level	0	10	10	10	0	0	30
Estimated Outlays	0	3	8	10	7	2	30
H.R. 5261, Treatment, Education, and Community Help to Combat Addiction Act of 2018:							
Authorization Level	0	4	4	4	4	4	20
Estimated Outlays	0	1	3	4	4	4	16
H.R. 5327, Comprehensive Opioid Recovery Centers Act of 2018:							
Authorization Level	0	10	10	10	10	10	50
Estimated Outlays	0	3	8	10	10	10	41
H.R. 5329, Poison Center Network Enhancement Act of 2018:							
Authorization Level	0	30	30	30	30	30	151
Estimated Outlays	0	12	25	29	29	29	125
H.R. 5353, Eliminating Opioid-Related Infectious Diseases Act of 2018:							
Authorization Level	0	40	40	40	40	40	200
Estimated Outlays	0	15	34	38	39	40	166
H.R. 5580, Surveillance and Testing of Opioids to Prevent Fentanyl Deaths Act of 2018:							
Authorization Level	30	30	30	30	30	0	120
Estimated Outlays	0	11	25	29	29	19	113
H.R. 5587, Peer Support Communities of Recovery Act:							
Authorization Level	0	15	15	15	15	15	75
Estimated Outlays	0	5	13	14	15	15	62

Annual amounts may not sum to totals because of rounding. * = between zero and $500,000.

H.R. 4684, the Ensuring Access to Quality Sober Living Act, would direct the Secretary of HHS to develop and disseminate best practices for organizations that operate housing designed for people recovering from substance use disorders. The bill would authorize a total of $3 million over the 2019–2021 period for that purpose. Based on historical spending patterns for similar activities, CBO estimates that implementing H.R. 4684 would cost $3 million over the 2019–2023 period.

H.R. 5102, the Substance Use Disorder Workforce Loan Repayment Act of 2018, would establish a loan repayment program for mental health professionals who practice in areas with few mental health providers or with high rates of death from overdose and would authorize $25 million per year over the 2019–2028 period for that purpose. Based on historical spending patterns for similar activities, CBO estimates that implementing H.R. 5102 would cost $100 million over the 2019–2023 period; the remaining amounts would be spent in years after 2023.

H.R. 5176, the Preventing Overdoses While in Emergency Rooms Act of 2018, would require the Secretary of HHS to develop protocols and a grant program for health care providers to address the needs of people who survive a drug overdose, and it would authorize $50 million in 2019 for that purpose. Based on historical spending patterns for similar activities, CBO estimates that implementing H.R. 5176 would cost $50 million over the 2019–2023 period.

H.R. 5197, the Alternatives to Opioids (ALTO) in the Emergency Department Act, would direct the Secretary of HHS to carry out a demonstration program for hospitals and emergency departments to develop alternative protocols for pain management that limit the use of opioids and would authorize $10 million annually in grants for fiscal years 2019 through 2021. Based on historical spending patterns for similar programs, CBO estimates that implementing H.R. 5197 would cost $30 million over the 2019–2023 period.

H.R. 5261, the Treatment, Education, and Community Help to Combat Addiction Act of 2018, would direct the Secretary of HHS to designate regional centers of excellence to improve the training of health professionals who treat substance use disorders. The bill would authorize $4 million annually for grants to those programs over the 2019–2023 period. Based on historical spending patterns for similar activities, CBO estimates that implementing H.R. 5261 would cost $16 million over the 2019–2023 period; the remaining amounts would be spent in years after 2023.

H.R. 5327, the Comprehensive Opioid Recovery Centers Act of 2018, would direct the Secretary of HHS to award grants to at least 10 providers that offer treatment services for people with opioid use disorder, and it would authorize $10 million per year over the 2019–2023 period for that purpose. Based on historical spending patterns for similar activities, CBO estimates that implementing H.R. 5327 would cost $41 million over the 2019–2023 period; the remaining amounts would be spent in years after 2023.

H.R. 5329, the Poison Center Network Enhancement Act of 2018, would reauthorize the poison control center toll-free number, national media campaign, and grant program under the Public Health Service Act. Among other actions, H.R. 5329 would increase the share of poison control center funding that could be provided by federal grants. The bill would authorize a total of about $30 million per year over the 2019–2023 period. Based on historical spending patterns for similar activities, CBO estimates that implementing H.R. 5329 would cost $125 million over the 2019–2023 period; the remaining amounts would be spent in years after 2023.

H.R. 5353, the Eliminating Opioid Related Infectious Diseases Act of 2018, would amend the Public Health Service Act by broadening the focus of surveillance and education programs from preventing and treating hepatitis C virus to preventing and treating infections associated with injection drug use. It would authorize $40 million per year over 2019–2023 period for that purpose. Based on historical spending patterns for similar activities, CBO estimates that implementing H.R. 5353 would cost $166 million over the 2019–2023 period; the remaining amounts would be spent in years after 2023.

H.R. 5580, the Surveillance and Testing of Opioids to Prevent Fentanyl Deaths Act of 2018, would establish a grant program for public health laboratories that conduct testing for fentanyl and other synthetic opioids. It also would direct the Centers for Disease Control and Prevention to expand its drug surveillance program, with a particular focus on collecting data on fentanyl. The bill would authorize a total of $30 million per year over the 2018–2022 period for those activities. Based on historical spending patterns for similar activities, CBO estimates that implementing H.R. 5580 would cost $113 million over the 2019–2023 period; the remaining amounts would be spent in years after 2023.

H.R. 5587, Peer Support Communities of Recovery Act, would direct the Secretary of HHS to award grants to nonprofit organizations that support community-based, peer-delivered support, including technical support for the establishment of recovery community organizations, independent, nonprofit groups led by people in recovery and their families. The bill would authorize $15 million per year for the 2019–2023 period. Based on historical spending patterns for similar activities, CBO estimates that implementing H.R. 5587 would cost $62 million over the 2019–2023 period; the remaining amounts would be spent in years after 2023.

Estimated Authorizations. Table 3 shows CBO's estimates of the appropriations that would be necessary to implement 19 of the bills. Spending would be subject to appropriation of those amounts.

H.R. 449, the Synthetic Drug Awareness Act of 2018, would require the Surgeon General to report to the Congress on the health effects of synthetic psychoactive drugs on children between the ages of 12 and 18. Based on spending patterns for similar activities, CBO estimates that implementing H.R. 449 would cost approximately $1 million over the 2019–2023 period.

H.R. 4005, the Medicaid Reentry Act, would direct the Secretary of HHS to convene a group of stakeholders to develop and report to the Congress on best practices for addressing issues related to health care faced by those returning from incarceration to their communities. The bill also would require the Secretary to issue a letter to state Medicaid directors about relevant demonstration projects. Based on an analysis of anticipated workload, CBO estimates that implementing H.R. 4005 would cost less than $500,000 over the 2018–2023 period.

H.R. 4275, the Empowering Pharmacists in the Fight Against Opioid Abuse Act, would require the Secretary of HHS to develop and disseminate materials for training pharmacists, health care practitioners, and the public about the circumstances under which a pharmacist may decline to fill a prescription. Based on historical spending patterns for similar activities, CBO estimates that costs to the federal government for the development and distribution of those materials would not be significant.

Table 3. Estimated Spending Subject to Appropriation for Bills with Estimated

	By fiscal year, in millions of dollars—						
	2018	2019	2020	2021	2022	2023	2019-2023
INCREASES IN SPENDING SUBJECT TO APPROPRIATION							
H.R. 449, Synthetic Drug Awareness Act of 2018:							
Estimated Authorization Level	0	*	*	*	0	0	1
Estimated Outlays	0	*	*	*	0	0	1
H.R. 4005, Medicaid Reentry Act:							
Estimated Authorization Level	*	*	0	0	0	0	*
Estimated Outlays	*	*	0	0	0	0	*
H.R. 4275, Empowering Pharmacists in the Fight Against Opioid Abuse Act:							
Estimated Authorization Level	0	*	*	*	*	*	*
Estimated Outlays	0	*	*	*	*	*	*
H.R. 5009, Jessie's Law:							
Estimated Authorization Level	0	*	*	*	*	*	*
Estimated Outlays	0	*	*	*	*	*	*
H.R. 5041, Safe Disposal of Unused Medication Act:							
Estimated Authorization Level	0	*	*	*	*	*	*
Estimated Outlays	0	*	*	*	*	*	*
H.R. 5272, Reinforcing Evidence-Based Standards Under Law in Treating Substance Abuse Act of 2018:							
Estimated Authorization Level	0	1	1	1	1	1	4
Estimated Outlays	0	1	1	1	1	1	4
H.R. 5333, Over-the-Counter Monograph Safety, Innovation, and Reform Act of 2018: [a]							
Food and Drug Administration:							
Collections from fees:							
Estimated Authorization Level	0	– 22	– 22	– 26	– 35	– 42	– 147
Estimated Outlays	0	– 22	– 22	– 26	– 35	– 42	– 147

Table 3. (Continued)

	By fiscal year, in millions of dollars—						
	2018	2019	2020	2021	2022	2023	2019-2023
Spending of fees:							
Estimated Authorization Level	0	22	22	26	35	42	147
Estimated Outlays	0	6	17	30	44	41	137
Net effect on FDA:							
Estimated Authorization Level	0	0	0	0	0	0	0
Estimated Outlays	0	– 17	– 6	4	9	*	– 10
Government Accountability Office:							
Estimated Authorization Level	0	0	0	0	0	*	*
Estimated Outlays	0	0	0	0	0	*	*
Total, H.R. 5333:							
Estimated Authorization Level	0	0	0	0	0	0	0
Estimated Outlays	0	– 17	– 6	4	9	*	– 10
H.R. 5473, Better Pain Management Through Better Data Act of 2018:							
Estimated Authorization Level	0	*	*	*	*	0	1
Estimated Outlays	0	*	*	*	*	*	1
H.R. 5483, Special Registration for Telemedicine Clarification Act of 2018:							
Estimated Authorization Level	0	*	*	*	*	*	*
Estimated Outlays	0	*	*	*	*	*	*
H.R. 5554, Animal Drug and Animal Generic Drug User Fee Amendments of 2018:							
Collections from fees:							
Animal drug fees	0	– 30	– 31	– 32	– 33	– 34	– 159
Generic animal drug fees	0	– 18	– 19	– 19	– 20	– 21	– 97
Total, Estimated Authorization Level	0	– 49	– 50	– 51	– 53	– 55	– 257

	By fiscal year, in millions of dollars—						
	2018	**2019**	**2020**	**2021**	**2022**	**2023**	**2019-2023**
Total, Estimated Outlays	0	– 49	– 50	– 51	– 53	– 55	– 257
Spending of fees:							
Animal drug fees	0	30	31	32	33	34	159
Generic animal drug fees	0	18	19	19	20	21	97
Total, Estimated Authorization Level	0	49	50	51	53	55	257
Total, Estimated Outlays	0	39	47	51	52	54	243
Net changes in fees:							
Estimated Authorization Level	0	0	0	0	0	0	0
Estimated Outlays	0	– 10	– 3	*	*	*	– 14
Other effects:							
Estimated Authorization Level	0	3	1	1	1	1	6
Estimated Outlays	0	2	1	1	1	1	6
Total, H.R. 5554:							
Estimated Authorization Level	0	3	1	1	1	1	6
Estimated Outlays	0	– 8	– 2	1	*	*	– 8
H.R. 5582, Abuse Deterrent Access Act of 2018:							
Estimated Authorization Level	0	0	*	0	0	0	*
Estimated Outlays	0	0	*	0	0	0	*
H.R. 5590, Opioid Addiction Action Plan Act:							
Estimated Authorization Level	*	*	*	*	*	*	2
Estimated Outlays	*	*	*	*	*	*	2
H.R. 5687, Securing Opioids and Unused Narcotics with Deliberate Disposal and Packaging Act of 2018:							
Estimated Authorization Level	0	*	*	*	*	*	*
Estimated Outlays	0	*	*	*	*	*	*
H.R. 5715, Strengthening Partnerships to Prevent Opioid Abuse Act:							
Estimated Authorization Level	0	2	2	2	2	2	9

Table 3. (Continued)

	By fiscal year, in millions of dollars—						
	2018	**2019**	**2020**	**2021**	**2022**	**2023**	**2019-2023**
Estimated Outlays	0	2	2	2	2	2	9
H.R. 5789, a bill to require the Secretary of Health and Human Services to issue guidance to improve care for infants with neonatal abstinence syndrome and their mothers, and to require the Comptroller General of the United States to conduct a study on gaps in Medicaid coverage for pregnant and postpartum women with substance use disorder:							
Estimated Authorization Level	0	2	0	0	0	0	2
Estimated Outlays	0	2	0	0	0	0	2
H.R. 5795, Overdose Prevention and Patient Safety Act:							
Estimated Authorization Level	0	1	0	0	0	0	1
Estimated Outlays	0	1	0	0	0	0	1
H.R. 5800, Medicaid IMD ADDITIONAL INFO Act:							
Estimated Authorization Level	0	1	0	0	0	0	1
Estimated Outlays	0	*	*	0	0	0	1
H.R. 5804, Post-Surgical Injections as an Opioid Alternative Act: [a]							
Estimated Authorization Level	0	0	0	0	1	1	1
Estimated Outlays	0	0	0	0	1	1	1
H.R. 5811, a bill to amend the Federal Food, Drug, and Cosmetic Act with respect to postapproval study requirements for certain controlled substances, and for other purposes:							
Estimated Authorization Level	0	*	*	*	*	*	*
Estimated Outlays	0	*	*	*	*	*	*

Annual amounts may not sum to totals because of rounding. * = between – $500,000 and $500,000.

[a] This bill also would affect mandatory spending (see Table 1).

H.R. 5009, Jessie's Law, would require HHS, in collaboration with outside experts, to develop best practices for displaying information about opioid use disorder in a patient's medical record. HHS also would be required to develop and disseminate written materials annually to health care providers about what disclosures could be made while still complying with federal laws that govern health care privacy. Based on spending patterns for similar activities, CBO estimates that implementing H.R. 5009 would have an insignificant effect on spending over the 2019–2023 period.

H.R. 5041, the Safe Disposal of Unused Medication Act, would require hospice programs to have written policies and procedures for the disposal of controlled substances after a patient's death. Certain licensed employees of hospice programs would be permitted to assist in the disposal of controlled substances that were lawfully dispensed. Using information from the Department of Justice (DOJ), CBO estimates that implementing the bill would cost less than $500,000 over the 2019–2023 period.

H.R. 5272, the Reinforcing Evidence-Based Standards Under Law in Treating Substance Abuse Act of 2018, would require the newly established National Mental Health and Substance Use Policy Laboratory to issue guidance to applicants for SAMHSA grants that support evidence-based practices. Using information from HHS about the historical cost of similar activities, CBO estimates that enacting this bill would cost approximately $4 million over the 2019–2023 period.

H.R. 5333, the Over-the-Counter Monograph Safety, Innovation, and Reform Act of 2018, would change the FDA's oversight of the commercial marketing of OTC medicines and authorize the collection and spending of fees through 2023 to cover the costs of expediting the FDA's administrative procedures for certain regulatory activities relating to OTC products. Under H.R. 5333, CBO estimates, the FDA would assess about $147 million in fees over the 2019–2023 period that could be collected and made available for obligation only to the extent and in the amounts provided in advance in appropriation acts. Because the FDA could spend those fees, CBO estimates that the estimated budget authority for collections and spending would offset each other exactly in each year, although CBO expects that spending initially would lag behind collections.

Assuming appropriation action consistent with the bill, CBO estimates that implementing H.R. 5333 would reduce net discretionary outlays by $10 million over the 2019–2023 period, primarily because of that lag. The bill also would require the Government Accountability Office to study exclusive market protections for certain qualifying OTC drugs authorized by the bill—a provision that CBO estimates would cost less than $500,000. (If enacted, H.R. 5333 also would affect mandatory spending; see Table 1.)

H.R. 5473, the Better Pain Management Through Better Data Act of 2018, would require that the FDA conduct a public meeting and issue guidance to industry addressing data collection and labeling for medical products that reduce pain while enabling the reduction, replacement, or avoidance of oral opioids. Using information from the agency, CBO estimates that implementing H.R. 5473 would cost about $1 million over the 2019–2023 period.

H.R. 5483, the Special Registration for Telemedicine Clarification Act of 2018, would direct DOJ, within one year of the bill's enactment, to issue regulations concerning the practice of telemedicine (for remote diagnosis and treatment of patients). Using information from DOJ, CBO estimates that implementing the bill would cost less than $500,000 over the 2019–2023 period.

H.R. 5554, the Animal Drug and Animal Generic Drug User Fee Amendments of 2018, would authorize the FDA to collect and spend fees to cover the cost of expedited approval for the development and marketing of certain drugs for use in animals. The legislation would extend through fiscal year 2023, and make several changes to, the FDA's existing approval processes and fee programs for brand-name and generic veterinary drugs, which expire at the end of fiscal year 2018. CBO estimates that implementing H.R. 5554 would reduce net discretionary outlays by $8 million over the 2019–2023 period, primarily because the spending of fees lags somewhat behind their collection.

Fees authorized under the bill would supplement funds appropriated to cover the FDA's cost of reviewing certain applications and investigational submissions for brand-name and generic drugs for use in animals. Those fees could be collected and made available for obligation only to the extent and in the amounts provided in advance in appropriation acts. Under H.R. 5554, CBO estimates, the FDA would assess about $257 million in fees over the 2019–2023 period. Because the FDA could spend those funds, CBO estimates that budget authority for collections and spending would offset each other exactly in each year. CBO estimates that the delay between collecting and spending fees under the reauthorized programs would reduce net discretionary outlays by $14 million over the 2019–2023 period, assuming appropriation actions consistent with the bill.

Enacting H.R. 5554 would increase the FDA's workload because the legislation would expand eligibility for conditional approval for certain drugs. The agency's administrative costs also would increase because of regulatory activities required by a provision concerning petitions for additives intended for use in animal food. H.R. 5554 also would require the FDA to publish guidance or produce regulations on a range of topics, transmit a report to the Congress, and hold public meetings. CBO expects that the costs associated with those activities would not be covered by fees, and it estimates that implementing such provisions would cost $6 million over the 2019–2023 period.

H.R. 5582, the Abuse Deterrent Access Act of 2018, would require the Secretary of HHS to report to the Congress on existing barriers to access to "abuse-deterrent opioid formulations" by Medicare Part C and D beneficiaries. Such formulations make the drugs more difficult to dissolve for injection, for example, and thus can impede their abuse. Assuming the availability of appropriated funds and based on historical spending patterns for similar activities, CBO estimates that implementing the legislation would cost less than $500,000 over the 2019–2023 period.

H.R. 5590, the Opioid Addiction Action Plan Act, would require the Secretary of HHS to develop an action plan by January 1, 2019, for increasing access to medication-assisted treatment among Medicare and Medicaid enrollees. The bill also would require HHS to convene a stakeholder meeting and issue a request for information within three months of enactment, and to submit a report to the Congress by June 1, 2019. Based on historical spending patterns for similar activities, CBO estimates that implementing H.R. 5590 would cost approximately $2 million over the 2019–2023 period.

H.R. 5687, the Securing Opioids and Unused Narcotics with Deliberate Disposal and Packaging Act of 2018, would permit the FDA to require certain packaging and disposal technologies, controls, or measures to mitigate the risk of abuse and misuse of drugs. Based on information from the FDA, CBO estimates that implementing H.R. 5687 would not significantly affect spending over the 2019–2023 period. This bill would also require that the GAO study the effectiveness and use of packaging technologies for controlled substances—a provision that CBO estimates would cost less than $500,000.

H.R. 5715, the Strengthening Partnerships to Prevent Opioid Abuse Act, would require the Secretary of HHS to establish a secure Internet portal to allow HHS, Medicare Advantage plans, and Medicare Part D plans to exchange information about fraud, waste, and abuse among providers and suppliers no later than two years after enactment. H.R. 5715 also would require organizations with Medicare Advantage contracts to submit information on investigations related to providers suspected of prescribing large volumes of opioids through a process established by the Secretary no later than January 2021. Based on historical spending patterns for similar activities, CBO estimates that implementing H.R. 5715 would cost approximately $9 million over the 2019–2023 period.

H.R. 5789, a bill to require the Secretary of Health and Human Services to issue guidance to improve care for infants with neonatal abstinence syndrome and their mothers, and to require the Comptroller General of the United States to conduct a study on gaps in Medicaid coverage for pregnant and postpartum women with substance use disorder, would direct the Secretary of HHS to issue guidance to states on best practices under Medicaid and CHIP for treating infants with neonatal abstinence syndrome. H.R. 5789 also would direct the Government Accountability Office to study Medicaid coverage for pregnant and postpartum women with substance use disorders. Based on information from HHS and historical spending patterns for similar activities, CBO estimates that enacting H.R. 5789 would cost approximately $2 million over the 2019–2023 period.

H.R. 5795, the Overdose Prevention and Patient Safety Act, would amend the Public Health Service Act so that requirements pertaining to the confidentiality and disclosure of medical records relating to substance use disorders align with the provisions of the Health Insurance Portability and Accountability Act of 1996. The bill would require the Office of the Secretary of HHS to issue regulations prohibiting discrimination based on data disclosed from such medical records, to issue regulations requiring covered entities to provide written notice of privacy practices, and to develop model training programs and materials for health care providers and patients and their families. Based on spending patterns for similar activities, CBO estimates that implementing H.R. 5795 would cost approximately $1 million over the 2019–2023 period.

H.R. 5800, Medicaid IMD ADDITIONAL INFO Act, would direct the Medicaid and CHIP Payment and Access Commission to study institutions for mental diseases in a representative sample of states. Based on information from the commission about the cost of similar work, CBO estimates that implementing H.R. 5800 would cost about $1 million over the 2019–2023 period.

H.R. 5804, the Post-Surgical Injections as an Opioid Alternative Act, would freeze the Medicare payment rate for certain analgesic injections provided in ambulatory surgical centers. The bill also would mandate two studies of Medicare coding and payments arising from enactment of this legislation. Based on the cost of similar activities, CBO estimates that those reports would cost $1 millionover the 2019–2023 period. (If enacted, H.R. 5804 also would affect mandatory spending; see Table 1.)

H.R. 5811, a bill to amend the Federal Food, Drug, and Cosmetic Act with respect to postapproval study requirements for certain controlled substances, and for other purposes, would allow the FDA to require that pharmaceutical manufacturers study certain drugs after they are approved to assess any potential reduction in those drugs' effectiveness for the conditions of use prescribed, recommended, or suggested in labeling. CBO anticipates that implementing H.R. 5811 would not significantly affect the FDA's costs over the 2019–2023 period.

Other Authorizations. The following nine bills would increase authorization levels, but CBO has not completed estimates of amounts. All authorizations would be subject to future appropriation action.

- H.R. 4284, Indexing Narcotics, Fentanyl, and Opioids Act of 2017
- H.R. 5002, Advancing Cutting Edge Research Act
- H.R. 5228, Stop Counterfeit Drugs by Regulating and Enhancing Enforcement Now Act (see Table 1 for an estimate of the revenue effects of H.R. 5228)
- H.R. 5752, Stop Illicit Drug Importation Act of 2018 (see Table 1 for an estimate of the revenue effects of H.R. 5752)
- H.R. 5799, Medicaid DRUG Improvement Act (see Table 1 for an estimate of the direct spending effects of H.R. 5799)
- H.R. 5801, Medicaid Providers and Pharmacists Are Required to Note Experiences in Record Systems to Help In-Need Patients (PARTNERSHIP) Act (see Table 1 for an estimate of the direct spending effects of H.R. 5801)
- H.R. 5806, 21st Century Tools for Pain and Addiction Treatments Act
- H.R. 5808, Medicaid Pharmaceutical Home Act of 2018 (see Table 1 for an estimate of the direct spending effects of H.R. 5808)
- H.R. 5812, Creating Opportunities that Necessitate New and Enhanced Connections That Improve Opioid Navigation Strategies Act (CONNECTIONS) Act

Pay-As-You-Go considerations: The Statutory Pay-As-You-Go Act of 2010 establishes budget-reporting and enforcement procedures for legislation affecting direct spending or revenues. Twenty-two of the bills discussed in this document contain direct spending or revenues and are subject to pay-as-you-go procedures. Details about the amount of direct spending and revenues in those bills can be found in Table 1.

Increase in long-term direct spending and deficits: CBO estimates that enacting H.R. 4998, the Health Insurance for Former Foster Youth Act, would increase net direct spending by more than $2.5 billion and on-budget deficits by more than $5 billion in at least one of the four consecutive 10-year periods beginning in 2029.

CBO estimates that none of the remaining 58 bills included in this estimate would increase net direct spending by more than $2.5 billion or on-budget deficits by more than $5 billion in any of the four consecutive 10-year periods beginning in 2029.

Mandates: One of the 59 bills included in this document, H.R. 5795, would impose both intergovernmental and private-sectormandates as defined in UMRA. CBO estimates that the costs of that bill's mandates on public and private entities would fall below UMRA's thresholds ($80 million and $160 million, respectively, for public-and private-sector entities in 2018, adjusted annually for inflation).

In addition, five bills would impose private-sector mandates as defined in UMRA. CBO estimates that the costs of the mandates in three of those bills (H.R. 5333, H.R. 5554, and H.R. 5811) would fall below the UMRA threshold. Because CBO does not know how federal agencies would implement new authority granted in the other two of those five bills, H.R. 5228 and 5687, CBO cannot determine whether the costs of their mandates would exceed the threshold.

For large entitlement grant programs, including Medicaid and CHIP, UMRA defines an increase in the stringency of conditions on states or localities as an intergovernmental mandate if the affected governments lack authority to offset those costs while continuing to provide required services. Because states possess significant flexibility to alter their responsibilities within Medicaid and CHIP, the requirements imposed by various bills in the markup on state administration of those programs would not constitute mandates as defined in UMRA.

Mandates Affecting Public and Private Entities

H.R. 5795, the Overdose Prevention and Patient Safety Act, would impose intergovernmental and private-sector mandates by requiring entities that provide treatment for substance use disorders to notify patients of their privacy rights and also to notify patients in the event that the confidentiality of their records is breached. In certain circumstances, H.R. 5795 also would prohibit public and private entities from denying entry to treatment on the basis of information in patient health records. Those requirements would either supplant or narrowly expand responsibilities under existing law, and compliance with them would not impose significant additional costs. CBO estimates that the costs of the mandates would fall below the annual thresholds established in UMRA.

Mandates Affecting Private Entities

Five bills included in this document would impose private-sector mandates:

H.R. 5228, the Stop Counterfeit Drugs by Regulating and En- hancing Enforcement Now Act, would require drug distributors to cease distributing any drug that the Secretary of HHS determines might present an imminent or substantial hazard to public health. CBO cannot determine what drugs could be subject to such an order nor can it determine how private entities would respond. Consequently, CBO cannot determine whether the aggregate cost of the mandate would exceed the annual threshold for private-sec- tor mandates.

H.R. 5333, the Over-the-Counter Monograph Safety, Innovation, and Reform Act of 2018, would require developers and manufacturers of OTC drugs to pay certain fees to the FDA. CBO estimates that about $30 million would be collected each year, on average, for a total of $147 million over the 2019–2023 period. Those amounts would not exceed the annual threshold for private-sector mandates in any year during that period.

H.R. 5554, the Animal Drug and Animal Generic Drug User Fee Amendments of 2018, would require developers and manufacturers of brand-name and generic veterinary drugs to pay application, product, establishment, and sponsor fees to the FDA. CBO estimates that about $51 million would be collected annually, on average, for a total of $257 million over the 2019–2023 period. Those amounts would not exceed the annual threshold for private-sector mandates in any year during that period.

H.R. 5687, the Securing Opioids and Unused Narcotics with Deliberate Disposal and Packaging Act of 2018, would permit the Secretary of HHS to require drug developers and manufacturers to implement new packaging and disposal technology for certain drugs. Based on information from the agency, CBO expects that the Secretary would use the new regulatory authority provided in the bill; however, it is uncertain how or when those requirements would be implemented. Consequently, CBO cannot determine whether the aggregate cost of the mandate would exceed the annual threshold for private entities.

H.R. 5811, a bill to amend the Federal Food, Drug, and Cosmetic Act with respect to postapproval study requirements for certain controlled substances, and for other purposes, would expand an existing mandate that requires drug developers to conduct postapproval studies or clinical trials for certain drugs. Under current law, in certain instances, the FDA can require studies or clinical trials after a drug has been approved. H.R. 5811 would permit the FDA to use that authority if the reduction in a drug's effectiveness meant that its benefits no longer outweighed its costs. CBO estimates that the incremental cost of the mandate would fall below the annual threshold established in UMRA because of the small number of drugs affected and the narrow expansion of the authority that exists under current law.

None of the remaining 53 bills included in this document would impose an intergovernmental or private-sector mandate.

Previous CBO estimate: On June 6, 2018, CBO issued an estimate for seven opioid-related bills ordered reported by the House Committee on Ways and Means on May 16, 2018. Two of those bills contain provisions that are identical or similar to the legislation ordered reported by the Committee on Energy and Commerce, and for those provisions, CBO's estimates are the same.

In particular, five bills listed in this estimate contain provisions that are identical or similar to those in several sections of H.R. 5773, the Preventing Addiction for Susceptible Seniors Act of 2018:

- H.R. 5675, which would require prescription drug plans to implement drug management programs, is identical to section 2 of H.R. 5773.
- H.R. 4841, regarding electronic prior authorization for prescriptions under Medicare's Part D, is similar to section 3 of H.R. 5773.
- H.R. 5715, which would mandate the creation of a new Internet portal to allow various stakeholders to exchange information, is identical to section 4 of H.R. 5773.
- H.R. 5684, which would expand medication therapy management, is the same as section 5 of H.R. 5773.
- H.R. 5716, regarding prescriber notification, is identical to section 6 of H.R. 5773.

In addition, in this estimate, a provision related to Medicare beneficiary education in H.R. 5686, the Medicare Clear Health Options in Care for Enrollees Act of 2018, is the same as a provision in section 2 of H.R. 5775, the Providing Reliable Options for Patients and Educational Resources Act of 2018, in CBO's estimate for the Committee on Ways and Means.

Estimate prepared by: Federal Costs: Rebecca Yip (Centers for Disease Control and Prevention), Mark Grabowicz (Drug Enforcement Agency), Julia Christensen, Ellen Werble (Food and Drug Administration), Emily King, Andrea Noda, Lisa Ramirez-Branum, Robert Stewart (Medicaid and Children's Health Insurance Program), Philippa Haven, Lara Robillard, Colin Yee, Rebecca Yip (Medicare), Philippa Haven (National Institutes of Health), Alice Burns, Andrea Noda (Office of the Secretary of the Department of Health and Human Services), Philippa Haven, Lori Housman, Emily King (Substance Abuse and Mental Health Services Administration, Health Resources and Services Administration); Federal Revenues: Jacob Fabian, Peter Huether, and Cecilia Pastrone; Fact Checking: Zachary Byrum and Kate Kelly; Mandates: Andrew Laughlin.

Estimate reviewed by: Tom Bradley, Chief, Health Systems and Medicare Cost Estimates Unit; Chad M. Chirico, Chief, Low-Income Health Programs and Prescription Drugs Cost Estimates Unit; Sarah Masi, Special Assistant for Health; Susan Willie, Chief, Mandates Unit; Leo Lex, Deputy Assistant Director for Budget Analysis; Theresa A. Gullo, Assistant Director for Budget Analysis.

Federal Mandates Statement

The Committee adopts as its own the estimate of Federal mandates prepared by the Director of the Congressional Budget Office pursuant to section 423 of the Unfunded Mandates Reform Act.

Statement of General Performance Goals and Objectives

Pursuant to clause 3(c)(4) of rule XIII, the general performance goal or objective of this legislation is to require prescription drug plan sponsors under the Medicare program to establish drug management programs for at-risk beneficiaries.

This requirement is currently voluntary for plans.

DUPLICATION OF FEDERAL PROGRAMS

Pursuant to clause 3(c)(5) of rule XIII, no provision of H.R. 5675 is known to be duplicative of another Federal program, including any program that was included in a report to Congress pursuant to section 21 of Public Law 111–139 or the most recent Catalog of Federal Domestic Assistance.

COMMITTEE COST ESTIMATE

Pursuant to clause 3(d)(1) of rule XIII, the Committee adopts as its own the cost estimate prepared by the Director of the Congressional Budget Office pursuant to section 402 of the Congressional Budget Act of 1974.

EARMARK, LIMITED TAX BENEFITS, AND LIMITED TARIFF BENEFITS

Pursuant to clause 9(e), 9(f), and 9(g) of rule XXI, the Committee finds that H.R. 5675 contains no earmarks, limited tax benefits, or limited tariff benefits.

DISCLOSURE OF DIRECTED RULE MAKINGS

Pursuant to section 3(i) of H. Res. 5, the Committee finds that H.R. 3331 contains no directed rule makings.

ADVISORY COMMITTEE STATEMENT

No advisory committees within the meaning of section 5(b) of the Federal Advisory Committee Act were created by this legislation.

APPLICABILITY TO LEGISLATIVE BRANCH

The Committee finds that the legislation does not relate to the terms and conditions of employment or access to public services or accommodations within the meaning of section 102(b)(3) of the Congressional Accountability Act.

SECTION-BY-SECTION ANALYSIS OF THE LEGISLATION

Section 1. Requiring Prescription Drug Plan Sponsors under Medicare to Establish Drug Management Programs for at Risk Beneficiaries

Section 1 would require prescription drug plan sponsors in Medicare to establish a drug management program for at-risk beneficiaries by plan year 2021.

CHANGES IN EXISTING LAW MADE BY THE BILL, AS REPORTED

In compliance with clause 3(e) of rule XIII of the Rules of the House of Representatives, changes in existing law made by the bill, as reported, are shown as follows (new matter is printed in italic and existing law in which no change is proposed is shown in roman):

SOCIAL SECURITY ACT

Title XVIII—Health Insurance for the Aged and Disabled

Part D—Voluntary Prescription Drug Benefit Program

Subpart 1—Part D Eligible Individuals and Prescription Drug Benefits: Beneficiary Protections for Qualified Prescription Drug Coverage

Sec. 1860D–4.

(a) Dissemination of Information.—

(1) General Information.—

(A) Application of MA Information.—A PDP sponsor shall disclose, in a clear, accurate, and standardized form to each enrollee with a prescription drug plan offered by the sponsor under this part at the time of enrollment and at least annually thereafter, the information described in section 1852(c)(1) relating to such plan, insofar as the Secretary determines appropriate with respect to benefits provided under this part, and including the information described in subparagraph (B).

(B) Drug Specific Information.—The information described in this subparagraph is information concerning the following:

(i) Access to specific covered part D drugs, including access through pharmacy networks.

(ii) How any formulary (including any tiered formulary structure) used by the sponsor functions, including a description of how a part D eligible individual may obtain information on the formulary consistent with paragraph (3).

(iii) Beneficiary cost-sharing requirements and how a part D eligible individual may obtain information on such requirements, including tiered or other copayment level applicable to each drug (or class of drugs), consistent with paragraph (3).

(iv) The medication therapy management program required under subsection (c).

(v) The drug management program for at-risk beneficiaries under subsection (c)(5).

(2) Disclosure Upon Request of General Coverage, Utilization, and Grievance Information.—Upon request of a part D eligible individual who is eligible to enroll in a prescription drug plan, the PDP sponsor offering such plan shall provide information similar (as determined by the Secretary) to the information described in subparagraphs (A), (B), and (C) of section 1852(c)(2) to such individual.

(3) Provision of Specific Information.—

(A) Response to Beneficiary Questions.—Each PDP sponsor offering a prescription drug plan shall have a mechanism for providing specific information on a timely basis to enrollees upon request. Such mechanism shall include access to information through the use of a toll-free telephone number and, upon request, the provision of such information in writing.

(B) Availability of Information on Changes in Formulary Through the Internet.—A PDP sponsor offering a prescription drug plan shall make available on a timely basis through an Internet website information on specific changes in the formulary under the plan (including changes to tiered or preferred status of covered part D drugs).

(4) Claims Information.—A PDP sponsor offering a prescription drug plan must furnish to each enrollee in a form easily understandable to such enrollees—

(A) an explanation of benefits (in accordance with section 1806(a) or in a comparable manner); and

(B) when prescription drug benefits are provided under this part, a notice of the benefits in relation to—

(i) the initial coverage limit for the current year; and

(ii) the annual out-of-pocket threshold for the cur- rent year.

Notices under subparagraph (B) need not be provided more often than as specified by the Secretary and notices under subparagraph (B)(ii) shall take into account the application of section 1860D–2(b)(4)(C) to the extent practicable, as specified by the Secretary.

(b) Access to Covered Part D Drugs.—

(1) Assuring Pharmacy Access.—

(A) Participation of Any Willing Pharmacy.—A prescription drug plan shall permit the participation of any pharmacy that meets the terms and conditions under the plan.

(B) Discounts Allowed for Network Pharmacies.— For covered part D drugs dispensed through in-network pharmacies, a prescription drug plan may, notwithstanding subparagraph (A), reduce coinsurance or copayments for part D eligible individuals enrolled in the plan below the level otherwise required. In no case shall such a reduction result in an increase in payments made by the Secretary under section 1860D–15 to a plan.

(C) Convenient Access for Network Pharmacies.—

(i) In General.—The PDP sponsor of the prescription drug plan shall secure the participation in its network of a sufficient number of pharmacies that dispense (other than by mail order) drugs directly to patients to ensure convenient access (consistent with rules established by the Secretary).

(ii) Application of Tricare Standards.—The Secretary shall establish rules for convenient access to in-network pharmacies under this subparagraph that are no less favorable to enrollees than the rules for convenient access to pharmacies included in the statement of work of solicitation (#MDA906–03–R–0002) of the Department of Defense under the TRICARE Retail Pharmacy (TRRx) as of March 13, 2003.

(iii) Adequate Emergency Access.—Such rules shall include adequate emergency access for enrollees.

(iv) Convenient Access in Long-Term Care Facilities.—Such rules may include standards with respect to access for enrollees who are residing in long-term care facilities and for pharmacies operated by the Indian Health Service, Indian tribes and tribal organizations, and urban Indian organizations (as defined in section 4 of the Indian Health Care Improvement Act).

(D) Level Playing Field.—Such a sponsor shall permit enrollees to receive benefits (which may include a 90-day supply of drugs or biologicals) through a pharmacy (other than a mail order pharmacy), with any differential in charge paid by such enrollees.

(E) Not Required to Accept Insurance Risk.—The terms and conditions under subparagraph (A) may not require participating pharmacies to accept insurance risk as a condition of participation.

(2) Use of Standardized Technology.—

(A) In General.—The PDP sponsor of a prescription drug plan shall issue (and reissue, as appropriate) such a card (or other technology) that may be used by an enrollee to assure access to negotiated prices under section 1860D–2(d).

(B) Standards.—

(i) In General.—The Secretary shall provide for the development, adoption, or recognition of standards relating to a standardized format for the card or other technology required under subparagraph (A). Such standards shall be compatible with part C of title XI and may be based on standards developed by an appropriate standard setting organization.

(ii) Consultation.—In developing the standards under clause (i), the Secretary shall consult with the National Council for Prescription Drug Programs and other standard setting organizations determined appropriate by the Secretary.

(iii) Implementation.—The Secretary shall develop, adopt, or recognize the standards under clause (i) by such date as the Secretary determines shall be sufficient to ensure that PDP sponsors utilize such standards beginning January 1, 2006.

(3) Requirements on Development and Application of Formularies.—If a PDP sponsor of a prescription drug plan uses a formulary (including the use of tiered cost-sharing), the following requirements must be met:

(A) Development and revision by a Pharmacy and Therapeutic (P&T) Committee.—

(i) In General.—The formulary must be developed and reviewed by a pharmacy and therapeutic committee. A majority of the members of such committee shall consist of individuals who are practicing physicians or practicing pharmacists (or both).

(ii) Inclusion of Independent Experts.—Such committee shall include at least one practicing physician and at least one practicing pharmacist, each of whom—

(I) is independent and free of conflict with respect to the sponsor and plan; and

(II) has expertise in the care of elderly or disabled persons.

(B) Formulary Development.—In developing and reviewing the formulary, the committee shall—

(i) base clinical decisions on the strength of scientific evidence and standards of practice, including assessing peer-reviewed medical literature, such as randomized clinical trials, pharmacoeconomic studies, out-comes research data, and on such other information as the committee determines to be appropriate; and

(ii) take into account whether including in the formulary (or in a tier in such formulary) particular covered part D drugs has therapeutic advantages in terms of safety and efficacy.

(C) Inclusion of Drugs in All Therapeutic Categories and Classes.—

(i) In General.—Subject to subparagraph (G), the formulary must include drugs within each therapeutic category and class of covered part D drugs, although not necessarily all drugs within such categories and classes.

(ii) Model Guidelines.—The Secretary shall request the United States Pharmacopeia to develop, in consultation with pharmaceutical benefit managers and other interested parties, a list of categories and classes that may be used by prescription drug plans under this paragraph and to revise such classification from time to time to reflect changes in therapeutic uses of covered part D drugs and the additions of new covered part D drugs.

(iii) Limitation on Changes in Therapeutic Classification.—The PDP sponsor of a prescription drug plan may not change the therapeutic categories and classes in a formulary other than at the beginning of each plan year except as the Secretary may permit to take into account new therapeutic uses and newly approved covered part D drugs.

(D) Provider and Patient Education.—The PDP sponsor shall establish policies and procedures to educate and inform health care providers and enrollees concerning the formulary.

(E) Notice Before Removing Drug from Formulary OR Changing Preferred or Tier Status of Drug.—Any removal of a covered part D drug from a formulary and any change in the preferred or tiered cost-sharing status of such a drug shall take effect only after appropriate notice is made available (such as under subsection (a)(3)) to the Secretary, affected enrollees, physicians, pharmacies, and pharmacists.

(F) Periodic Evaluation of Protocols.—In connection with the formulary, the sponsor of a prescription drug plan shall provide for the periodic evaluation and analysis of treatment protocols and procedures.

(G) Required Inclusion of Drugs in Certain Categories and Classes.—

(i) Formulary Requirements.—

(I) In General.—Subject to subclause (II), a PDP sponsor offering a prescription drug plan shall be required to include all covered part D drugs in the categories and classes identified by the Secretary under clause (ii)(I).

(II) Exceptions.—The Secretary may establish exceptions that permit a PDP sponsor offering a prescription drug plan to exclude from its formulary a particular covered part D drug in a category or class that is otherwise required to be included in the formulary under subclause (I) (or to otherwise limit access to such a drug, including through prior authorization or utilization management).

(ii) Identification of Drugs in Certain Categories and Classes.—

(I) in General.—Subject to clause (iv), the Secretary shall identify, as appropriate, categories and classes of drugs for which the Secretary determines are of clinical concern.

(II) Criteria.—The Secretary shall use criteria established by the Secretary in making any determination under subclause (I).

(iii) Implementation.—The Secretary shall establish the criteria under clause (ii)(II) and any exceptions under clause (i)(II) through the promulgation of a regulation which includes a public notice and comment period.

(iv) Requirement for Certain Categories and Classes Until Criteria Established.—Until such time as the Secretary establishes the criteria under clause (ii)(II) the following categories and classes of drugs shall be identified under clause (ii)(I):

(I) Anticonvulsants.

(II) Antidepressants.

(III) Antineoplastics.

(IV) Antipsychotics.

(V) Antiretrovirals.

(VI) Immunosuppressants for the treatment of transplant rejection.

(H) Use of Single, Uniform Exceptions and Appeals Process.—Notwithstanding any other provision of this part, each PDP sponsor of a prescription drug plan shall— (i) use a single, uniform exceptions and appeals process (including, to the extent the Secretary determines feasible, a single, uniform model form for use under such process) with respect to the determination of prescription drug coverage for an enrollee under the plan; and

(ii) provide instant access to such process by enrollees through a toll-free telephone number and an Internet website.

© Cost and Utilization Management; Quality Assurance; Medication Therapy Management Program.—

(1) In General.—The PDP sponsor shall have in place, directly or through appropriate arrangements, with respect to covered part D drugs, the following:

(A) A cost-effective drug utilization management program, including incentives to reduce costs when medically appropriate, such as through the use of multiple source drugs (as defined in section 1927(k)(7)(A)(i)).

(B) Quality assurance measures and systems to reduce medication errors and adverse drug interactions and improve medication use.

(C) A medication therapy management program described in paragraph (2).

(D) A program to control fraud, abuse, and waste.

(E) A utilization management tool to prevent drug abuse (as described in paragraph (6)(A)).

(F) With respect to plan years beginning on or after January 1, 2021, a drug management program for at-risk beneficiaries described in paragraph (5).

Nothing in this section shall be construed as impairing a PDP sponsor from utilizing cost management tools (including differential payments) under all methods of operation.

(2) Medication Therapy Management Program.—

(A) Description.—

(i) In General.—A medication therapy management program described in this paragraph is a program of drug therapy management that may be furnished by a pharmacist and that is designed to assure, with respect to targeted beneficiaries described in clause (ii), that covered part D drugs under the prescription drug plan are appropriately used to optimize therapeutic outcomes through improved medication use, and to reduce the risk of adverse events, including adverse drug interactions. Such a program may distinguish between services in ambulatory and institutional settings.

(ii) Targeted Beneficiaries Described.—Targeted beneficiaries described in this clause are part D eligible individuals who—

(I) have multiple chronic diseases (such as diabetes, asthma, hypertension, hyperlipidemia, and congestive heart failure);

(II) are taking multiple covered part D drugs; and

(III) are identified as likely to incur annual costs for covered part D drugs that exceed a level specified by the Secretary.

(B) Elements.—Such program may include elements that promote—

(i) enhanced enrollee understanding to promote the appropriate use of medications by enrollees and to reduce the risk of potential adverse events associated with medications, through beneficiary education, counseling, and other appropriate means;

(ii) increased enrollee adherence with prescription medication regimens through medication refill reminders, special packaging, and other compliance programs and other appropriate means; and

(iii) detection of adverse drug events and patterns of overuse and underuse of prescription drugs.

(C) Required Interventions.—For plan years beginning on or after the date that is 2 years after the date of the enactment of the Patient Protection and Affordable Care Act, prescription drug plan sponsors shall offer medication therapy management services to targeted beneficiaries described in subparagraph (A)(ii) that include, at a minimum, the following to increase adherence to prescription medications or other goals deemed necessary by the Secretary:

(i) An annual comprehensive medication review furnished person-to-person or using telehealth technologies (as defined by the Secretary) by a licensed pharmacist or other qualified provider. The comprehensive medication review—

(I) shall include a review of the individual's medications and may result in the creation of a recommended medication action plan or other actions in consultation with the individual and with input from the prescriber to the extent necessary and practicable; and

(II) shall include providing the individual with a written or printed summary of the results of the review.

The Secretary, in consultation with relevant stakeholders, shall develop a standardized format for the action plan under subclause (I) and the summary under subclause (II).

(ii) Follow-up interventions as warranted based on the findings of the annual medication review or the targeted medication enrollment and which may be provided person-to-person or using telehealth technologies (as defined by the Secretary).

(D) Assessment.—The prescription drug plan sponsor shall have in place a process to assess, at least on a quarterly basis, the medication use of individuals who are at risk but not enrolled in the medication therapy management program, including individuals who have experienced a transition in care, if the prescription drug plan sponsor has access to that information.

(E) Automatic Enrollment with Ability to Opt-Out.— The prescription drug plan sponsor shall have in place a process to—

(i) subject to clause (ii), automatically enroll targeted beneficiaries described in subparagraph (A)(ii), including beneficiaries identified under subparagraph (D), in the medication therapy management program required under this subsection; and

(ii) permit such beneficiaries to opt-out of enrollment in such program.

(E) Development of Program in Cooperation with Licensed Pharmacists.—Such program shall be developed in cooperation with licensed and practicing pharmacists and physicians.

(F) Coordination with Care Management Plans.—The Secretary shall establish guidelines for the coordination of any medication therapy management program under this paragraph with respect to a targeted beneficiary with any care management plan established with respect to such beneficiary under a chronic care improvement program under section 1807.

(G) Considerations in Pharmacy Fees.—The PDP sponsor of a prescription drug plan shall take into account, in establishing fees for pharmacists and others providing services under such plan, the resources used, and time required to, implement the medication therapy management program under this paragraph. Each such sponsor shall disclose to the Secretary upon request the amount of any such management or dispensing fees. The provisions of section 1927(b)(3)(D) apply to information disclosed under this subparagraph.

(3) Reducing Wasteful Dispensing of Outpatient Prescription Drugs in Long-Term Care Facilities.—The Secretary shall require PDP sponsors of prescription drug plans to utilize

specific, uniform dispensing techniques, as determined by the Secretary, in consultation with relevant stakeholders (including representatives of nursing facilities, residents of nursing facilities, pharmacists, the pharmacy industry (including retail and long-term care pharmacy), prescription drug plans, MA–PD plans, and any other stakeholders the Secretary determines appropriate), such as weekly, daily, or automated dose dispensing, when dispensing covered part D drugs to enrollees who reside in a long-term care facility in order to reduce waste associated with 30-day fills.

(4) Requiring Valid Prescriber National Provider Identifiers on Pharmacy Claims.—

(A) In General.—For plan year 2016 and subsequent plan years, the Secretary shall require a claim for a covered part D drug for a part D eligible individual enrolled in a prescription drug plan under this part or an MA–PD plan under part C to include a prescriber National Provider Identifier that is determined to be valid under the procedures established under subparagraph (B)(i).

(B) Procedures.—

(i) Validity of Prescriber National Provider Identifiers.—The Secretary, in consultation with appropriate stakeholders, shall establish procedures for determining the validity of prescriber National Provider Identifiers under subparagraph (A).

(ii) Informing Beneficiaries of Reason for Denial.—The Secretary shall establish procedures to ensure that, in the case that a claim for a covered part D drug of an individual described in subparagraph (A) is denied because the claim does not meet the requirements of this paragraph, the individual is properly informed at the point of service of the reason for the denial.

(C) Report.—Not later than January 1, 2018, the Inspector General of the Department of Health and Human Services shall submit to Congress a report on the effectiveness of the procedures established under subparagraph (B)(i).

(5) Drug Management Program for at-Risk Beneficiaries.—

(A) Authority to Establish.—A PDP sponsor may *(and for plan years beginning on or after January 1, 2021, a PDP sponsor shall)* establish a drug management program for at-risk beneficiaries under which, subject to subparagraph (B), the PDP sponsor may, in the case of an at-risk beneficiary for prescription drug abuse who is an enrollee in a prescription drug plan of such PDP sponsor, limit such beneficiary's access to coverage for frequently abused drugs under such plan to frequently abused drugs that are prescribed for such beneficiary by one or more prescribers selected under subparagraph (D), and dispensed for such beneficiary by one or more pharmacies selected under such subparagraph.

(B) Requirement for Notices.—

(i) In General.—A PDP sponsor may not limit the access of an at-risk beneficiary for prescription drug abuse to coverage for frequently abused drugs under a prescription drug plan until such sponsor—

(I) provides to the beneficiary an initial notice described in clause (ii) and a second notice described in clause (iii); and

(II) verifies with the providers of the beneficiary that the beneficiary is an at-risk beneficiary for prescription drug abuse.

(ii) Initial Notice.—An initial notice described in this clause is a notice that provides to the beneficiary—

(I) notice that the PDP sponsor has identified the beneficiary as potentially being an at-risk beneficiary for prescription drug abuse;

(II) information describing all State and Federal public health resources that are designed to address prescription drug abuse to which the beneficiary has access, including mental health services and other counseling services;

(III) notice of, and information about, the right of the beneficiary to appeal such identification under subsection (h) and the option of an automatic escalation to external review;

(IV) a request for the beneficiary to submit to the PDP sponsor preferences for which prescribers and pharmacies the beneficiary would prefer the PDP sponsor to select under subparagraph (D) in the case that the beneficiary is identified as an at-risk beneficiary for prescription drug abuse as described in clause (iii)(I);

(V) an explanation of the meaning and consequences of the identification of the beneficiary as potentially being an at-risk beneficiary for prescription drug abuse, including an explanation of the drug management program established by the PDP sponsor pursuant to subparagraph (A);

(VI) clear instructions that explain how the beneficiary can contact the PDP sponsor in order to submit to the PDP sponsor the preferences described in subclause (IV) and any other communications relating to the drug management program for at-risk beneficiaries established by the PDP sponsor; and

(VII) contact information for other organizations that can provide the beneficiary with assistance regarding such drug management program (similar to the information provided by the Secretary in other standardized notices provided to part D eligible individuals enrolled in prescription drug plans under this part).

(iii) Second Notice.—A second notice described in this clause is a notice that provides to the beneficiary notice—

(I) that the PDP sponsor has identified the beneficiary as an at-risk beneficiary for prescription drug abuse;

(II) that such beneficiary is subject to the requirements of the drug management program for at-risk beneficiaries established by such PDP sponsor for such plan;

(III) of the prescriber (or prescribers) and pharmacy (or pharmacies) selected for such individual under subparagraph (D);

(IV) of, and information about, the beneficiary's right to appeal such identification under subsection (h) and the option of an automatic escalation to external review;

(V) that the beneficiary can, in the case that the beneficiary has not previously submitted to the PDP sponsor preferences for which prescribers and pharmacies the beneficiary would prefer the PDP sponsor select under subparagraph (D), submit such preferences to the PDP sponsor; and

(VI) that includes clear instructions that explain how the beneficiary can contact the PDP sponsor.

(iv) Timing of Notices.—

(I) In General.—Subject to subclause (II), a second notice described in clause (iii) shall be provided to the beneficiary on a date that is not less than 30 days after an initial notice described in clause (ii) is provided to the beneficiary.

(II) Exception.—In the case that the PDP sponsor, in conjunction with the Secretary, determines that concerns identified through rulemaking by the

Secretary regarding the health or safety of the beneficiary or regarding significant drug diversion activities require the PDP sponsor to provide a second notice described in clause (iii) to the beneficiary on a date that is earlier than the date described in subclause (I), the PDP sponsor may provide such second notice on such earlier date.

(C) At-Risk Beneficiary for Prescription Drug Abuse.—

(i) In General.—For purposes of this paragraph, the term "at-risk beneficiary for prescription drug abuse" means a part D eligible individual who is not an exempted individual described in clause (ii) and—

(I) who is identified as such an at-risk beneficiary through the use of clinical guidelines that indicate misuse or abuse of prescription drugs described in subparagraph (G) and that are developed by the Secretary in consultation with PDP sponsors and other stakeholders, including individuals entitled to benefits under part A or enrolled under part B, advocacy groups representing such individuals, physicians, pharmacists, and other clinicians, retail pharmacies, plan sponsors, entities delegated by plan sponsors, and biopharmaceutical manufacturers; or

(II) with respect to whom the PDP sponsor of a prescription drug plan, upon enrolling such individual in such plan, received notice from the Secretary that such individual was identified under this paragraph to be an at-risk beneficiary for prescription drug abuse under the prescription drug plan in which such individual was most recently previously enrolled and such identification has not been terminated under subparagraph (F).

(ii) EXEMPTED INDIVIDUAL DESCRIBED.—An exempted individual described in this clause is an individual who—

(I) receives hospice care under this title;

(II) is a resident of a long-term care facility, of a facility described in section 1905(d), or of another facility for which frequently abused drugs are dispensed for residents through a contract with a single pharmacy; or

(III) the Secretary elects to treat as an exempted individual for purposes of clause (i).

(iii) Program Size.—The Secretary shall establish policies, including the guidelines developed under clause (i)(I) and the exemptions under clause (ii)(III), to ensure that the population of enrollees in a drug management program for at-risk beneficiaries operated by a prescription drug plan can be effectively managed by such plans.

(iv) Clinical Contact.—With respect to each at-risk beneficiary for prescription drug abuse enrolled in a prescription drug plan offered by a PDP sponsor, the PDP sponsor shall contact the beneficiary's providers who have prescribed frequently abused drugs regarding whether prescribed medications are appropriate for such beneficiary's medical conditions.

(D) Selection of Prescribers and Pharmacies.—

(i) In General.—With respect to each at-risk beneficiary for prescription drug abuse enrolled in a prescription drug plan offered by such sponsor, a PDP sponsor shall, based on the preferences submitted to the PDP sponsor by the beneficiary pursuant toclauses (ii)(IV) and (iii)(V) of subparagraph (B) (except as otherwise provided in this subparagraph) select—

(I) one, or, if the PDP sponsor reasonably determines it necessary to provide the beneficiary with reasonable access under clause (ii), more than one, individual who is authorized to prescribe frequently abused drugs (referred to in this paragraph as a "prescriber") who may write prescriptions for such drugs for such beneficiary; and

(II) one, or, if the PDP sponsor reasonably determines it necessary to provide the beneficiary with reasonable access under clause (ii), more than one, pharmacy that may dispense such drugs to such beneficiary.

For purposes of subclause (II), in the case of a pharmacy that has multiple locations that share real-time electronic data, all such locations of the pharmacy shall collectively be treated as one pharmacy.

(ii) Reasonable Access.—In making the selections under this subparagraph—

(I) a PDP sponsor shall ensure that the beneficiary continues to have reasonable access to frequently abused drugs (as defined in subparagraph (G)), taking into account geographic location, beneficiary preference, impact on costsharing, and reasonable travel time; and

(II) a PDP sponsor shall ensure such access (including access to prescribers and pharmacies with respect to frequently abused drugs) in the case of individuals with multiple residences, in the case of natural disasters and similar situations, and in the case of the provision of emergency services.

(iii) Beneficiary Preferences.—If an at-risk beneficiary for prescription drug abuse submits preferences for which in-network prescribers and pharmacies the beneficiary would prefer the PDP sponsor select in response to a notice under subparagraph (B), the PDP sponsor shall—

(I) review such preferences;

(II) select or change the selection of prescribers and pharmacies for the beneficiary based on such preferences; and

(III) inform the beneficiary of such selection or change of selection.

(iv) Exception Regarding Beneficiary Preferences.—In the case that the PDP sponsor determines that a change to the selection of prescriber or pharmacy under clause (iii)(II) by the PDP sponsor is contributing or would contribute to prescription drug abuse or drug diversion by the beneficiary, the PDP sponsor may change the selection of prescriber or pharmacy for the beneficiary without regard to the preferences of the beneficiary described in clause (iii). If the PDP sponsor changes the selection pursuant to the preceding sentence, the PDP sponsor shall provide the beneficiary with—

(I) at least 30 days written notice of the change of selection; and

(II) a rationale for the change.

(v) Confirmation.—Before selecting a prescriber or pharmacy under this subparagraph, a PDP sponsor must notify the prescriber and pharmacy that the beneficiary involved has been identified for inclusion in the drug management program for at-risk beneficiaries and that the prescriber and pharmacy has been selected as the beneficiary's designated prescriber and pharmacy.

(E) TERMINATIONS AND APPEALS.—The identification of an individual as an at-risk beneficiary for prescription drug abuse under this paragraph, a coverage determination made under a drug management program for at-risk beneficiaries, the selection of prescriber or pharmacy under subparagraph (D), and information to be shared under subparagraph (I), with respect to such individual, shall be subject to reconsideration and appeal under subsection (h) and the option of an automatic escalation to external review to the extent provided by the Secretary.

(F) TERMINATION OF IDENTIFICATION.—

(i) IN GENERAL.—The Secretary shall develop standards for the termination of identification of an individual as an at-risk beneficiary for prescription drug abuse under this paragraph. Under such standards such identification shall terminate as of the earlier of—

(I) the date the individual demonstrates that the individual is no longer likely, in the absence of the restrictions under this paragraph, to be an at-risk beneficiary for prescription drug abuse described in subparagraph (C)(i); and

(II) the end of such maximum period of identification as the Secretary may specify.

(ii) Rule Of Construction.—Nothing in clause (i) shall be construed as preventing a plan from identifying an individual as an at-risk beneficiary for prescription drug abuse under subparagraph (C)(i) after such termination on the basis of additional information on drug use occurring after the date of notice of such termination.

(G) Frequently Abused Drug.—For purposes of this subsection, the term "frequently abused drug" means a drug that is a controlled substance that the Secretary determines to be frequently abused or diverted.

(H) Data Disclosure.—

(i) Data on Decision to Impose Limitation.—In the case of an at-risk beneficiary for prescription drug abuse (or an individual who is a potentially at-risk beneficiary for prescription drug abuse) whose access to coverage for frequently abused drugs under a prescription drug plan has been limited by a PDP sponsor under this paragraph, the Secretary shall establish rules and procedures to require the PDP sponsor to disclose data, including any necessary individually identifiable health information, in a form and manner specified by the Secretary, about the decision to impose such limitations and the limitations imposed by the sponsor under this part.

(ii) Data To Reduce Fraud, Abuse, And Waste.— The Secretary shall establish rules and procedures to require PDP sponsors operating a drug management program for at-risk beneficiaries under this paragraph to provide the Secretary with such data as the Secretary determines appropriate for purposes of identifying patterns of prescription drug utilization for plan enrollees that are outside normal patterns and that may indicate fraudulent, medically unnecessary, or unsafe use.

(I) Sharing of Information for Subsequent Plan Enrollments.—The Secretary shall establish procedures under which PDP sponsors who offer prescription drug plans shall share information with respect to individuals who are at-risk beneficiaries for prescription drug abuse (or individuals who are potentially at-risk beneficiaries for prescription drug abuse) and enrolled in a prescription drug plan and who subsequently disenroll from such plan and enroll in another prescription drug plan offered by another PDP sponsor.

(J) Privacy Issues.—Prior to the implementation of the rules and procedures under this paragraph, the Secretary shall clarify privacy requirements, including requirements under the regulations promulgated pursuant to section 264(c) of the Health Insurance Portability and Accountability Act of 1996 (42 U.S.C. 1320d–2 note), related to the sharing of data under subparagraphs (H) and (I) by PDP sponsors. Such clarification shall provide that the sharing of such data shall be considered to be protected health information in accordance with the requirements of the regulations promulgated pursuant to such section 264(c).

(K) Education.—The Secretary shall provide education to enrollees in prescription drug plans of PDP sponsors and providers regarding the drug management program for at-risk beneficiaries described in this paragraph, including education—

(i) provided by Medicare administrative contractors through the improper payment outreach and education program described in section 1874A(h); and

(ii) through current education efforts (such as State health insurance assistance programs described in subsection (a)(1)(A) of section 119 of the Medicare Improvements for Patients and Providers Act of 2008 (42 U.S.C. 1395b–3 note)) and materials directed toward such enrollees.

(L) Application Under MA–PD Plans.—Pursuant to section 1860D–21(c)(1), the provisions of this paragraph apply under part D to MA organizations offering MA–PD plans to MA eligible individuals in the same manner as such provisions apply under this part to a PDP sponsor offering a prescription drug plan to a part D eligible individual.

(M) CMS Compliance Review.—The Secretary shall ensure that existing plan sponsor compliance reviews and audit processes include the drug management programs for at-risk beneficiaries under this paragraph, including appeals processes under such programs.

(6) Utilization Management Tool to Prevent Drug Abuse.—

(A) In General.—A tool described in this paragraph is any of the following:

(i) A utilization tool designed to prevent the abuse of frequently abused drugs by individuals and to prevent the diversion of such drugs at pharmacies.

(ii) Retrospective utilization review to identify—

(I) individuals that receive frequently abused drugs at a frequency or in amounts that are not clinically appropriate; and

(II) providers of services or suppliers that may facilitate the abuse or diversion of frequently abused drugs by beneficiaries.

(iii) Consultation with the contractor described in subparagraph (B) to verify if an individual enrolling in a prescription drug plan offered by a PDP sponsor has been previously identified by another PDP sponsor as an individual described in clause (ii)(I).

(B) Reporting.—A PDP sponsor offering a prescription drug plan (and an MA organization offering an MA–PD plan) in a State shall submit to the Secretary and the Medicare drug integrity contractor with which the Secretary has entered into a contract under section 1893 with respect to such State a report, on a monthly basis, containing information on—

(i) any provider of services or supplier described in subparagraph (A)(ii)(II) that is identified by such plan sponsor (or organization) during the 30-day period before such report is submitted; and

(ii) the name and prescription records of individuals described in paragraph (5)(C).

(C) CMS Compliance Review.—The Secretary shall ensure that plan sponsor compliance reviews and program audits biennially include a certification that utilization management tools under this paragraph are in compliance with the requirements for such tools.

(6) Providing Prescription Drug Plans with Parts A and B Claims Data to Promote the Appropriate Use of Medications and Improve Health Outcomes.—

(A) Process.—Subject to subparagraph (B), the Secretary shall establish a process under which a PDP sponsor of a prescription drug plan may submit a request for the Secretary to provide the sponsor, on a periodic basis and in an electronic format, beginning in plan year 2020, data described in subparagraph (D) with respect to enrollees in such plan. Such data shall be provided without regard to whether such enrollees are described in clause (ii) of paragraph (2)(A).

(B) Purposes.—A PDP sponsor may use the data provided to the sponsor pursuant to subparagraph (A) for any of the following purposes:

(i) To optimize therapeutic outcomes through improved medication use, as such phrase is used in clause (i) of paragraph (2)(A).

(ii) To improving care coordination so as to prevent adverse health outcomes, such as preventable emergency department visits and hospital readmissions.

(iii) For any other purpose determined appropriate by the Secretary.

(C) Limitations on Data Use.—A PDP sponsor shall not use data provided to the sponsor pursuant to subparagraph (A) for any of the following purposes:

(i) To inform coverage determinations under this part.

(ii) To conduct retroactive reviews of medically accepted indications determinations.

(iii) To facilitate enrollment changes to a different prescription drug plan or an MA–PD plan offered by the same parent organization.

(iv) To inform marketing of benefits.

(v) For any other purpose that the Secretary determines is necessary to include in order to protect the identity of individuals entitled to, or enrolled for, benefits under this title and to protect the security of personal health information.

(D) Data Described.—The data described in this clause are standardized extracts (as determined by the Secretary) of claims data under parts A and B for items and services furnished under such parts for time periods specified by the Secretary. Such data shall include data as current as practicable.

(d) Consumer Satisfaction Surveys.—In order to provide for comparative information under section 1860D–1(c)(3)(A)(v), the Secretary shall conduct consumer satisfaction surveys with respect to PDP sponsors and prescription drug plans in a manner similar to the manner such surveys are conducted for MA organizations and MA plans under part C.

(e) Electronic Prescription Program.—

(1) Application of Standards.—As of such date as the Secretary may specify, but not later than 1 year after the date of promulgation of final standards under paragraph (4)(D), prescriptions and other information described in paragraph (2)(A) for covered part D drugs prescribed for part D eligible individuals that are transmitted electronically shall be transmitted only in accordance with such standards under an electronic prescription drug program that meets the requirements of paragraph (2).

(2) Program Requirements.—Consistent with uniform standards established under paragraph (3)—

(A) Provision of Information to Prescribing Health Care Professional and Dispensing Pharmacies and Pharmacists.—An electronic prescription drug program shall provide for the electronic transmittal to the prescribing health care professional and to the dispensing pharmacy and pharmacist of the prescription and information on eligibility and benefits (including the drugs included in the applicable formulary, any tiered formulary structure, and any requirements for prior authorization) and of the following information with respect to the prescribing and dispensing of a covered part D drug:

(i) Information on the drug being prescribed or dispensed and other drugs listed on the medication history, including information on drug-drug interactions, warnings or cautions, and, when indicated, dosage adjustments.

(ii) Information on the availability of lower cost, therapeutically appropriate alternatives (if any) for the drug prescribed.

(B) Application to Medical History Information.—Effective on and after such date as the Secretary specifies and after the establishment of appropriate standards to carry out this subparagraph, the program shall provide for the electronic transmittal in a manner similar to the manner under subparagraph (A) of information that relates to the medical history concerning the individual and related to a covered part D drug being prescribed or dispensed, upon request of the professional or pharmacist involved.

(C) Limitations.—Information shall only be disclosed under subparagraph (A) or (B) if the disclosure of such information is permitted under the Federal regulations (concerning the privacy of individually identifiable health information) promulgated under section 264(c) of the Health Insurance Portability and Accountability Act of 1996.

(D) Timing.—To the extent feasible, the information exchanged under this paragraph shall be on an interactive, real-time basis.

(3) Standards.—

(A) In General.—The Secretary shall provide consistent with this subsection for the promulgation of uniform standards relating to the requirements for electronic prescription drug programs under paragraph (2).

(B) Objectives.—Such standards shall be consistent with the objectives of improving—

(i) patient safety;

(ii) the quality of care provided to patients; and

(iii) efficiencies, including cost savings, in the delivery of care.

(C) Design Criteria.—Such standards shall—

(i) be designed so that, to the extent practicable, the standards do not impose an undue administrative burden on prescribing health care professionals and dispensing pharmacies and pharmacists;

(ii) be compatible with standards established under part C of title XI, standards established under subsection (b)(2)(B)(i), and with general health information technology standards; and

(iii) be designed so that they permit electronic exchange of drug labeling and drug listing information maintained by the Food and Drug Administration and the National Library of Medicine.

(D) Permitting Use of Appropriate Messaging.—Such standards shall allow for the messaging of information only if it relates to the appropriate prescribing of drugs, including quality assurance measures and systems referred to in subsection (c)(1)(B).

(E) Permitting Patient Designation of Dispensing Pharmacy.—

(i) In General.—Consistent with clause (ii), such standards shall permit a part D eligible individual to designate a particular pharmacy to dispense a prescribed drug.

(ii) No Change in Benefits.—Clause (i) shall not be construed as affecting—

(I) the access required to be provided to pharmacies by a prescription drug plan; or

(II) the application of any differences in benefits or payments under such a plan based on the pharmacy dispensing a covered part D drug.

(4) Development, Promulgation, and Modification of Standards.—

(A) Initial Standards.—Not later than September 1, 2005, the Secretary shall develop, adopt, recognize, or modify initial uniform standards relating to the requirements for electronic prescription drug programs described in paragraph (2) taking into consideration the recommendations (if any) from the National Committee on Vital and Health Statistics (as established under section 306(k) of the Public Health Service Act (42 U.S.C. 242k(k))) under subparagraph (B).

(B) Role OF NCVHS.—The National Committee on Vital and Health Statistics shall develop recommendations for uniform standards relating to such requirements in consultation with the following:

(i) Standard setting organizations (as defined in section 1171(8))

(ii) Practicing physicians.

(iii) Hospitals.

(iv) Pharmacies.

(v) Practicing pharmacists.

(vi) Pharmacy benefit managers.

(vii) State boards of pharmacy.

(viii) State boards of medicine.

(ix) Experts on electronic prescribing.

(x) Other appropriate Federal agencies.

(C) Pilot Project to Test Initial Standards.—

(i) In General.—During the 1-year period that begins on January 1, 2006, the Secretary shall conduct a pilot project to test the initial standards developed under subparagraph (A) prior to the promulgation of the final uniform standards under subparagraph (D) in order to provide for the efficient implementation of the requirements described in paragraph (2).

(ii) Exception.—Pilot testing of standards is not required under clause (i) where there already is adequate industry experience with such standards, as determined by the Secretary after consultation with effected standard setting organizations and industry users.

(iii) Voluntary Participation of Physicians and Pharmacies.—In order to conduct the pilot project under clause (i), the Secretary shall enter into agreements with physicians, physician groups, pharmacies, hospitals, PDP sponsors, MA organizations, and other appropriate entities under which health care professionals electronically transmit prescriptions to dispensing pharmacies and pharmacists in accordance with such standards.

(iv) Evaluation and Report.—

(I) Evaluation.—The Secretary shall conduct an evaluation of the pilot project conducted under clause (i).

(II) Report to Congress.—Not later than April 1, 2007, the Secretary shall submit to Congress a report on the evaluation conducted under subclause (I).

(D) Final Standards.—Based upon the evaluation of the pilot project under subparagraph (C)(iv)(I) and not later than April 1, 2008, the Secretary shall promulgate uniform standards relating to the requirements described in paragraph (2).

(5) Relation to State Laws.—The standards promulgated under this subsection shall supersede any State law or regulation that—

(A) is contrary to the standards or restricts the ability to carry out this part; and

(B) pertains to the electronic transmission of medication history and of information on eligibility, benefits, and prescriptions with respect to covered part D drugs under this part.

(6) Establishment of Safe Harbor.—The Secretary, in consultation with the Attorney General, shall promulgate regulations that provide for a safe harbor from sanctions under paragraphs (1) and (2) of section 1128B(b) and an exception to the prohibition under subsection (a)(1) of section 1877 with respect to the provision of nonmonetary remuneration (in the form of hardware, software, or information technology and training services) necessary and used solely to receive and transmit electronic prescription information in accordance with the standards promulgated under this subsection—

(A) in the case of a hospital, by the hospital to members of its medical staff;

(B) in the case of a group practice (as defined in section 1877(h)(4)), by the practice to prescribing health care professionals who are members of such practice; and

(C) in the case of a PDP sponsor or MA organization, by the sponsor or organization to pharmacists and pharmacies participating in the network of such sponsor or organization, and to prescribing health care professionals.

(f) Grievance Mechanism.—Each PDP sponsor shall provide meaningful procedures for hearing and resolving grievances between the sponsor (including any entity or individual through which the sponsor provides covered benefits) and enrollees with prescription drug plans of the sponsor under this part in accordance with section 1852(f).

(g) Coverage Determinations and Reconsiderations.—

(1) Application of Coverage Determination and Reconsideration Provisions.—A PDP sponsor shall meet the requirements of paragraphs (1) through (3) of section 1852(g) with respect to covered benefits under the prescription drug plan it offers under this part in the same manner as such requirements apply to an MA organization with respect to benefits it offers under an MA plan under part C.

(2) Request for a Determination for the Treatment of Tiered Formulary Drug.—In the case of a prescription drug plan offered by a PDP sponsor that provides for tiered costsharing for drugs included within a formulary and provides lower cost-sharing for preferred drugs included within the formulary, a part D eligible individual who is enrolled in the plan may request an exception to the tiered cost-sharing structure. Under such an exception, a nonpreferred drug could be covered under the terms applicable for preferred drugs if the prescribing physician determines that the preferred drug for treatment of the same condition either would not be as effective for the individual or would have adverse effects for the individual or both. A PDP sponsor shall have an exceptions process under this paragraph consistent with guidelines established by the Secretary for making a determination with respect to such a request. Denial of such an exception shall be treated as a coverage denial for purposes of applying subsection (h).

(h) Appeals.—

(1) In general.—Subject to paragraph (2), a PDP sponsor shall meet the requirements of paragraphs (4) and (5) of section 1852(g) with respect to benefits (including a determination related to the application of tiered cost-sharing described in subsection (g)(2)) in a manner similar (as determined by the Secretary) to the manner such requirements apply to an MA organization with respect to benefits under the original medicare fee-for-service program option it offers under an MA plan under part C. In applying this paragraph only the part D eligible individual shall be entitled to bring such an appeal.

(2) Limitation in cases on nonformulary determinations.—A part D eligible individual who is enrolled in a prescription drug plan offered by a PDP sponsor may appeal under paragraph (1) a determination not to provide for coverage of a covered part D drug that is not on the formulary under the plan only if the prescribing physician determines that all covered part D drugs on any tier of the formulary for treatment of the same condition would not be as effective for the individual as the nonformulary drug, would have adverse effects for the individual, or both.

(3) Treatment of nonformulary determinations.—If a PDP sponsor determines that a plan provides coverage for a covered part D drug that is not on the formulary of the plan, the drug shall be treated as being included on the formulary for purposes of section 1860D–2(b)(4)(C)(i).

(i) Privacy, Confidentiality, and Accuracy of Enrollee Records.—The provisions of section 1852(h) shall apply to a PDP sponsor and prescription drug plan in the same manner as it applies to an MA organization and an MA plan.

(j) Treatment of Accreditation.—Subparagraph (A) of section 1852(e)(4) (relating to treatment of accreditation) shall apply to a PDP sponsor under this part with respect to the following requirements, in the same manner as it applies to an MA organization with respect to the requirements in subparagraph (B) (other than clause (vii) thereof) of such section:

(1) Subsection (b) of this section (relating to access to covered part D drugs).

(2) Subsection (c) of this section (including quality assurance and medication therapy management).

(3) Subsection (i) of this section (relating to confidentiality and accuracy of enrollee records).

(k) Public Disclosure of Pharmaceutical Prices for Equivalent Drugs.—

(1) In general.—A PDP sponsor offering a prescription drug plan shall provide that each pharmacy that dispenses a covered part D drug shall inform an enrollee of any differential between the price of the drug to the enrollee and the price of the lowest priced generic covered part D drug under the plan that is therapeutically equivalent and bioequivalent and available at such pharmacy.

2. Timing of notice.—

(A) In general.—Subject to subparagraph (B), the information under paragraph (1) shall be provided at the time of purchase of the drug involved, or, in the case of dispensing by mail order, at the time of delivery of such drug.

(B) Waiver.—The Secretary may waive subparagraph

(A) in such circumstances as the Secretary may specify.

(l) Requirements with Respect to Sales and Marketing Activities.—The following provisions shall apply to a PDP sponsor (and the agents, brokers, and other third parties representing such sponsor) in the same manner as such provisions apply to a Medicare Advantage organization (and the agents, brokers, and other third parties representing such organization):

(1) The prohibition under section 1851(h)(4)(C) on conducting activities described in section 1851(j)(1).

(2) The requirement under section 1851(h)(4)(D) to conduct activities described in section 1851(j)(2) in accordance with the limitations established under such subsection.

(3) The inclusion of the plan type in the plan name under section 1851(h)(6).

(4) The requirements regarding the appointment of agents and brokers and compliance with State information requests under subparagraphs (A) and (B), respectively, of section 1851(h)(7).

Congress of the United States

House of Representatives

COMMITTEE ON ENERGY AND COMMERCE

2125 RAYBURN HOUSE OFFICE BUILDING

WASHINGTON, DC 20515-6115

Majority (202) 225-2927

Minority (202) 225-3641

June 7, 2018

The Honorable Kevin Brady

Chairman

Committee on Ways and Means

II 02 Longworth House Office Building

Washington, DC 20515

Dear Chairman Brady:

On May 9 and 17, 2018, the Committee on Energy and Commerce ordered favorably reported over 50 bills to address the opioid epidemic facing communities across our nation. Several of the bills were also referred to the Committee on Ways and Means.

I ask that the Committee on Ways and Means not insist on its referral of the following bills so that they may he scheduled for consideration by the Majority Leader:

- H.R. 1925, At-Risk Youth Medicaid Protection Act of2017;
- H.R. 3331, To amend title XI of the Social Security Act to promote testing of incentive payments for behavioral health providers for adoption and use of certified electronic health record technology;
- H.R. 3528, Every Prescription Conveyed Securely Act;
- H.R. 4841, Standardizing Electronic Prior Authorization for Safe Prescribing Act of 2018;
- H.R.5582, Abuse Deterrent Access Act of2018;
- H.R.5590, Opioid Addiction Action Plan Act;
- H.R. 5603, Access to Telehealth Services for Opioid Use Disorder;
- H.R. 5605, Advancing High Quality Treatment for Opioid Use Disorders in Medicare Act;
- II.R. 5675, To amend title XVIII of the Social Security Act to require prescription drug plan sponsors under the Medicare program to establish drug management programs for at-risk beneficiaries;
- H.R. 5684, Protecting Seniors from Opioid Abuse Act;
- H.R. 5685, Medicare Opioid Safety Education Act;
- H.R. 5686, Medicare Clear Health Options in Care for Enrollees (Cl!OICE) Act;
- H.R. 5715, Strengthening Partnerships to Prevent Opioid Abuse Act;
- H.R. 5716, Commit to Opioid Medical Prescriber Accountability and Safety for Seniors (COMPASS) Act;
- H.R. 5796, Responsible Education Achieves Care and Healthy Outcomes for Users' Treatment (REACH OUT) Act of2018;
- H.R. 5798, Opioid Screening and Chronic Pain Management Alternatives for Seniors Act;
- H.R. 5804, Post-Surgical Injections as an Opioid Alternative Act; and
- H.R. 5809, Postoperative Opioid Prevention Act of 2018.

This concession in no way affects your jurisdiction over the subject matter of these bills. and it will not serve as precedent for future referrals. In addition, should a conference on the bills be necessary, I would support your request to have the Committee on Ways and Means on the conference committee. Finally, I would be pleased to include this letter and your response in the bill reports and the Congressional Record.

Thank you for your consideration of my request and tor the extraordinary cooperation shown by you and your staff over matters of shared jurisdiction. I look forward to further opportunities to work with you this Congress.

Sincerely,

Greg Walden
Chairman

Congress of the United States
U.S. House of Representatives
COMMITTEE ON WAYS AND MEANS
1102 LONGWORTH HOUSE OFFICE BUILDING
(202) 225-3625
Washington, DC 20515-0348
http://waysandmeans.house.gov

June 8, 2018

The Honorable Greg Walden
Chairman
Committee on Energy and Commerce
2125 Rayburn House Office Building
Washington, DC 20515

Dear Chairman Walden,

Thank you for your letter concerning several bills favorably reported out of the Committee on Energy and Commerce to address the opioid epidemic and which the Committee on Ways and Means was granted an additional referral.

As a result of your having consulted with us on provisions within these bills that fall within the Rule X jurisdiction of the Committee on Ways and Means, I agree to waive formal consideration of the following bills so that they may move expeditiously to the floor:

- H.R. 1925, At-Risk Youth Medicaid Protection Act of 2017;
- H.R. 3331, To amend title Xl of the Social Security Act to promote testing of incentive payments for behavioral health providers for adoption and use of certified electronic health record technology;
- H.R. 3528, Every Prescription Conveyed Securely Act;
- H.R. 4841, Standardizing Electronic Prior Authorization for Safe Prescribing Act of 2018;
- H.R. 5582, Abuse Deterrent Access Act of2018;
- H.R.5590, Opioid Addiction Action Plan Act;
- H.R. 5603, Access to Telehealth Services for Opioid Use Disorder;
- H.R. 5605, Advancing High Quality Treatment for Opioid Use Disorders in Medicare Act;
- H.R. 5675, To amend title XVlll of the Social Security Act to require prescription drug plan sponsors under the Medicare program to establish drug management programs for at-risk beneficiaries;
- H.R. 5684, Protecting Seniors from Opioid Abuse Act;
- H.R. 5685, Medicare Opioid Safety Education Act;
- H.R. 5686, Medicare Clear Health Options in Care for Enrollees (CHOICE) Act;
- H.R. 5715, Strengthening Partnerships to Prevent Opioid Abuse Act;
- H.R. 5716, Commit to Opioid Medical Prescriber Accountability and Safety for Seniors (COMPASS) Act;
- H.R. 5796, Responsible Education Achieves Care and Healthy Outcomes for Users· Treatment (REACH OUT) Act of2018;
- H.R. 5798, Opioid Screening and Chronic Pain Management Altematives for Seniors Act;

- H.R. 5804, Post-Surgical Injections as an Opioid Alternative Act; and
- H.R. 5809, Postoperative Opioid Prevention Act of 2018.

The Committee on Ways and Means takes this action with the mutual understanding that we do not waive any jurisdiction over the subject matter contained in this or similar legislation, and the Committee will be appropriately consulted and involved as the bill or similar legislation moves forward so that we may address any remaining issues that fall within our jurisdiction. The Committee also reserves the right to seek appointment of an appropriate number of conferees to any House-Senate conference involving this or similar legislation and requests your support for such a request.

Finally, I would appreciate your commitment to include this exchange of letters in the bill reports and the Congressional Record.

Sincerely,

Kevin Brady
Chairman

cc: The Honorable Paul Ryan, Speaker
The Honorable Richard E. Neal
The Honorable Frank Pallone
Thomas J. Wickham, Jr., Parliamentarian

INDEX

A

abuse, vii, viii, x, 33, 53, 54, 55, 125, 127, 128, 129, 130, 131, 132, 133, 134, 137, 142, 143, 144, 145, 146, 147, 151, 154, 160, 161, 163, 166, 171, 172, 173, 176, 179, 183, 184, 199, 224, 251, 252, 270, 278, 285
access, viii, ix, xi, 7, 8, 9, 12, 13, 18, 22, 57, 58, 61, 64, 69, 71, 75, 78, 79, 85, 89, 96, 98, 100, 101, 102, 104, 116, 123, 126, 127, 130, 131, 134, 135, 138, 139, 147, 149, 150, 154, 156, 157, 159, 160, 161, 163, 164, 165, 166, 167, 168, 169, 184, 213, 236, 251, 261, 262, 263, 264, 265, 268, 270, 272, 275, 276, 280, 283, 290, 295
adolescents, 202, 203, 205, 207, 210
adults, xi, 52, 56, 114, 119, 182, 192, 202, 203, 205, 207, 210, 214, 215, 216, 217, 218, 219, 220, 222, 230, 233
advancement, 11, 29, 36, 72, 75
advancements, 8, 56, 64, 75, 90, 116, 120, 121, 122
adverse effects, 293, 294
adverse event, 271
advocacy, 56, 98, 119, 167, 168, 278
age, x, 178, 201, 202, 203, 204, 205, 206, 207, 208, 209, 217, 218, 219, 220, 224, 229, 230
agencies, x, 53, 130, 138, 140, 157, 162, 165, 166, 167, 176, 177, 179, 187, 191, 194, 227, 228, 255, 291
aging population, xi, 213
antidepressants, 202, 207, 214, 218, 219
antipsychotic, 233
antipsychotic drugs, 233
appropriations, ix, 126, 153, 155, 156, 157, 158, 159, 160, 239, 244
assessment, 22, 28, 30, 31, 42, 76, 102, 103, 198, 237, 238
at-risk beneficiaries, viii, 223, 224, 232, 236, 259, 261, 263, 270, 275, 276, 277, 279, 281, 282, 283, 284, 285, 297, 299

B

beneficiaries, viii, 76, 223, 224, 232, 234, 236, 240, 251, 259, 261, 263, 270, 271,

273, 275, 276, 277, 279, 281, 282, 283, 284, 285, 297, 299
benefits, 10, 19, 23, 64, 75, 93, 102, 103, 184, 257, 260, 262, 263, 264, 265, 278, 287, 288, 290, 292, 293, 294
beta blocker, 214, 219, 221
biologics, vii, 2, 4, 7, 12, 13, 16, 17, 23, 32, 33, 64, 69, 83, 85, 90, 95, 99
biomarkers, 4, 6, 21, 27, 28, 36, 41, 42, 45, 56, 70, 71, 77, 80, 85, 89, 93, 96, 103, 118
biotechnology, 78, 121, 166
blood, 27, 41, 48, 121, 210
blood pressure, 41, 48
budget deficit, 228, 255

C

cancer, 33, 56, 57, 61, 63, 65, 68, 69, 72, 74, 99, 106, 122, 123, 195
caregivers, 23, 66, 87, 92, 184
central nervous system, 127, 202, 205, 207
challenges, 13, 46, 62, 63, 64, 74, 75, 90, 105, 138, 162, 224
chemical, 153, 154, 183, 192
children, 52, 56, 57, 114, 119, 192, 198, 202, 203, 205, 207, 210, 230, 233, 244
classification, 208, 220, 221, 267
clinical trials, 3, 6, 17, 18, 29, 36, 56, 58, 59, 62, 71, 72, 87, 91, 102, 103, 109, 110, 115, 257, 267
collaboration, 28, 62, 67, 69, 75, 84, 121, 152, 160, 249
commercial, x, 40, 176, 180, 191, 192, 198, 249
community, 6, 9, 26, 33, 48, 98, 119, 120, 152, 164, 180, 181, 183, 192, 244
compliance, 53, 139, 168, 185, 234, 256, 261, 271, 284, 286, 296
confidentiality, 135, 253, 256, 295
Congress, iv, viii, ix, 1, 2, 3, 4, 5, 6, 7, 9, 12, 13, 24, 25, 34, 35, 51, 55, 58, 63, 64, 75, 76, 81, 85, 94, 97, 98, 99, 105, 107, 108, 109, 117, 119, 120, 121, 122, 123, 127, 128, 130, 137, 138, 155, 156, 163, 168, 223, 226, 244, 251, 260, 275, 292, 298
consumer advocates, 7, 79
consumer protection, 132
controlled substances, viii, 125, 126, 129, 130, 131, 133, 139, 143, 144, 145, 146, 148, 149, 151, 152, 161, 163, 164, 168, 169, 171, 181, 182, 183, 185, 187, 188, 194, 227, 233, 234, 235, 236, 240, 248, 249, 252, 253, 257
controlled trials, 109
coordination, 28, 33, 42, 67, 75, 273, 286
cost, 36, 77, 82, 87, 90, 91, 108, 129, 135, 140, 147, 155, 158, 223, 226, 228, 230, 234, 237, 241, 242, 243, 244, 249, 250, 251, 252, 253, 256, 257, 260, 262, 266, 268, 270, 288, 289, 293, 294
cures, 3, 5, 8, 10, 47, 57, 79, 95, 97, 98, 105, 110

D

data analysis, 91
data collection, 4, 6, 77, 87, 140, 160, 250
data set, 233
data sharing, vii, ix, 126, 131, 135, 136, 137, 147, 152, 165, 166
data transfer, 135
database, viii, ix, 126, 134, 139, 152, 169, 208, 220
Department of Defense, 155, 163, 265
Department of Health and Human Services, 11, 34, 128, 132, 138, 155, 157, 201, 225, 227, 229, 259, 274
Department of Justice, 129, 130, 137, 142, 148, 151, 152, 154, 157, 159, 168, 172, 249

disclosure, 134, 170, 171, 253, 288
diseases, 3, 5, 16, 19, 25, 26, 27, 38, 47, 48, 49, 52, 55, 56, 57, 63, 64, 69, 76, 79, 92, 99, 101, 115, 118, 122, 253
disorder, 210, 233, 235, 236, 237, 243, 248, 249, 252
doctors, 34, 38, 43, 48, 146
drug abuse, viii, x, 125, 127, 128, 131, 134, 146, 166, 172, 270, 283
drug history, 136
drug interaction, 144, 148, 270, 271, 288
drug safety, 13, 22, 29, 30, 58, 70, 72, 89
drug therapy, 270
drug treatment, 117, 133
drug-addicted individuals, viii, 125, 131
drugs, vii, viii, x, xi, 2, 3, 4, 5, 7, 8, 9, 10, 11, 12, 13, 14, 16, 17, 18, 19, 21, 22, 25, 26, 35, 36, 37, 39, 41, 46, 47, 48, 52, 54, 55, 56, 57, 58, 59, 61, 62, 64, 65, 67, 68, 69, 71, 72, 73, 74, 76, 79, 84, 86, 90, 95, 99, 105, 106, 109, 111, 113, 114, 115, 119, 120, 121, 125, 127, 128, 129, 132, 133, 140, 143, 145, 149, 154, 162, 163, 176, 182, 183, 184, 187, 189, 190, 191, 193, 194, 195, 197, 198, 202, 205, 206, 207, 208, 214, 215, 217, 218, 219, 220, 221, 227, 233, 234, 235, 237, 238, 250, 251, 252, 253, 256, 257, 262, 263, 264, 265, 267, 268, 269, 270, 271, 274, 275, 279, 280, 283, 285, 287, 288, 289, 292, 293, 294, 295

E

economic competitiveness, 99
economic downturn, 146
ecosystem, 7, 105, 121
education, 150, 161, 167, 198, 237, 243, 258, 271, 284
educational materials, 177, 197, 198
emergency, 150, 165, 242, 265, 280, 286
employees, 66, 78, 81, 117, 249
enforcement, vii, viii, 126, 127, 129, 130, 131, 132, 134, 136, 138, 139, 140, 141, 142, 144, 146, 147, 148, 150, 151, 152, 163, 166, 167, 168, 169, 172, 175, 176, 179, 183, 187, 188, 190, 192, 194, 232, 238, 254, 256, 259
enrollment, 91, 143, 150, 234, 262, 272, 273, 287
environment, 44, 62, 74, 110, 190
environmental effects, 189
environmental impact, 190
Environmental Protection Agency, 175, 176, 179, 190
epidemic, viii, 125, 127, 128, 130, 143, 162, 225, 227, 296, 298
evidence, ix, 3, 5, 6, 11, 19, 24, 25, 27, 30, 38, 42, 45, 56, 57, 58, 59, 62, 67, 69, 71, 72, 73, 75, 77, 80, 87, 89, 96, 103, 106, 107, 109, 110, 111, 126, 141, 143, 145, 147, 148, 168, 181, 193, 224, 236, 249, 266
evidence-based practices, 249
evidentiary standards, 28
expertise, 31, 38, 39, 41, 48, 74, 77, 80, 82, 91, 96, 100, 104, 266

F

federal agency, x, 176
federal government, ix, x, 126, 127, 130, 151, 165, 230, 233, 244
federal hiring, 37, 74
federal law, 179, 182, 249
federal regulations, 185
financial, 11, 32, 78, 80, 81, 84, 100, 104, 130, 239
financial oversight, 11
financial planning, 32
financial stability, 80
financial support, 130

fiscal year, 43, 231, 232, 237, 241, 242, 245, 246, 247, 248, 250
Food and Drug Administration (FDA), v, vii, 1, 2, 3, 4, 5, 6, 7, 8, 9, 11, 12, 13, 14, 15, 16, 17, 18, 19, 20, 21, 22, 23, 24, 25, 26, 27, 28, 29, 30, 31, 32, 33, 34, 35, 36, 37, 38, 39, 46, 47, 48, 50, 51, 53, 54, 55, 56, 58, 59, 61, 62, 63, 64, 65, 66, 67, 68, 69, 70, 71, 72, 73, 74, 75,76, 77, 78, 79, 80, 81, 82, 83, 84, 85, 86, 87, 88, 89, 90, 91, 92, 93, 94, 95, 96, 97, 98, 99, 100, 101, 102, 103, 104, 105, 106, 107, 108, 109, 110, 111, 112, 113, 115, 116, 117, 118, 119, 120, 121, 122, 123, 130, 137, 175, 176, 177, 179, 181, 182, 184, 185, 186, 187, 189, 190, 191, 193, 197, 198, 199, 227, 232, 234, 238, 245, 246, 249, 250, 251, 252, 253, 256, 257, 259, 289
fraud, 137, 164, 224, 252, 270
funding, 14, 26, 62, 66, 72, 75, 80, 120, 121, 123, 135, 136, 141, 152, 155, 156, 157, 158, 159, 160, 234, 236, 243
funds, ix, 66, 75, 90, 126, 138, 139, 141, 153, 155, 156, 158, 159, 161, 165, 166, 172, 234, 250, 251

G

grant programs, 130, 159, 160, 255
grants, vii, ix, 48, 126, 130, 131, 137, 141, 151, 152, 153, 155, 157, 159, 161, 227, 237, 242, 243, 244, 249
guidance, 26, 28, 29, 30, 38, 42, 53, 54, 66, 67, 71, 87, 88, 89, 90, 91, 92, 93, 94, 101, 102, 103, 109, 135, 137, 197, 199, 248, 249, 250, 251, 252
guidelines, vii, x, 29, 62, 73, 106, 107, 135, 201, 273, 278, 279, 293

H

health, vii, ix, x, xi, 8, 24, 25, 30, 52, 54, 55, 56, 58, 75, 79, 87, 89, 119, 120, 121, 123, 126, 127, 128, 130, 131, 132, 136, 138, 140, 141, 142, 150, 160, 162, 164, 166, 167, 169, 170, 180, 183, 184, 198, 201, 208, 209, 213, 220, 221, 222, 228, 230, 231, 235, 236, 239, 242, 244, 249, 253, 256, 268, 278, 283, 284, 286, 287, 288, 289, 291, 292, 293, 297, 299
health care, x, xi, 8, 79, 89, 119, 120, 121, 127, 128, 138, 141, 142, 162, 164, 166, 167, 170, 183, 184, 198, 213, 220, 222, 235, 242, 244, 249, 253, 268, 288, 289, 291, 292, 293
health care professionals, 235, 289, 291, 292, 293
health care programs, 164
health care system, 167, 220
health condition, xi, 208, 209, 213, 221
health effects, 244
health information, vii, x, 126, 127, 130, 131, 151, 159, 160, 164, 166, 167, 169, 170, 283, 284, 287, 289
health insurance, 284
health needs, vii, x, 61, 64, 201
health practitioners, 136
heart disease, 48, 209, 219, 221
heart failure, 121
heroin, vii, x, 127, 128, 129, 131, 144, 147, 165, 172, 173, 178
heroin abuse, vii, 129, 131, 147, 172, 173
hiring, 8, 31, 36, 37, 38, 56, 62, 75, 78, 83, 84, 96, 104
history, 48, 85, 86, 132, 288, 292
House of Representatives, viii, 1, 11, 63, 78, 97, 118, 178, 226, 261
human, 14, 26, 29, 31, 35, 36, 45, 61, 63, 79, 81, 82, 83, 92, 95, 98, 100, 104, 105, 136, 190

human health, 61, 63, 190
human resources, 83

I

identification, viii, 109, 125, 131, 154, 157, 276, 277, 278, 281, 282
improvements, 8, 11, 19, 28, 51, 52, 77, 78, 97, 120, 122
individuals, viii, 109, 115, 125, 128, 129, 131, 143, 163, 164, 185, 193, 198, 224, 235, 236, 264, 266, 271, 272, 276, 278, 280, 283, 284, 285, 287
industry, vii, 2, 4, 7, 9, 11, 12, 13, 19, 22, 24, 25, 27, 28, 29, 32, 44, 46, 47, 55, 56, 71, 76, 77, 79, 84, 89, 92, 94, 95, 97, 101, 102, 107, 108, 109, 111, 117, 120, 121, 137, 166, 169, 250, 274, 291
information exchange, 136, 137, 289
information sharing, ix, 126, 130, 136, 137, 138, 163, 171
information technology, 13, 292
initiation, 82, 138, 144, 163
injections, 237, 253
institutions, 78, 229, 233, 253
integration, 30, 31, 96, 100, 138, 160
interoperability, vii, ix, x, 112, 126, 127, 130, 131, 137, 138, 139, 147, 152, 164, 171
intervention, viii, 41, 67, 125, 131
investment, 3, 6, 9, 25, 76, 121
issues, ix, 21, 22, 39, 83, 105, 110, 112, 117, 127, 130, 138, 169, 187, 244, 300

J

jurisdiction, 298, 299, 300

L

law enforcement, viii, x, 126, 127, 129, 130, 131, 132, 134, 136, 138, 139, 140, 141, 142, 146, 147, 150, 151, 152, 163, 166, 167, 169, 183, 187, 188, 192, 194
leadership, 8, 42, 55, 67, 118, 120
legislation, ix, 2, 5, 10, 52, 55, 115, 117, 121, 126, 128, 136, 137, 141, 157, 166, 172, 225, 226, 227, 228, 229, 237, 238, 240, 250, 251, 253, 254, 258, 259, 261, 300
local government, 151, 179

M

management, viii, 11, 27, 31, 74, 80, 104, 163, 185, 209, 222, 223, 224, 232, 236, 237, 240, 258, 259, 261, 263, 268, 270, 271, 272, 273, 275, 276, 277, 279, 281, 282, 283, 284, 286, 295, 297, 299
marketing, 15, 18, 21, 27, 29, 53, 90, 192, 238, 249, 250, 287
materials, 101, 192, 197, 244, 249, 253, 284
Medicaid, 134, 143, 144, 145, 150, 164, 225, 227, 229, 230, 231, 233, 234, 238, 239, 244, 245, 248, 251, 252, 253, 254, 255, 259, 297, 299
medical, 3, 5, 7, 8, 9, 18, 19, 26, 28, 30, 33, 44, 46, 47, 50, 59, 63, 71, 72, 74, 79, 83, 84, 90, 92, 96, 97, 100, 103, 104, 105, 106, 110, 111, 112, 114, 119, 120, 121, 122, 129, 130, 131, 133, 134, 141, 146, 147, 150, 152, 167, 178, 249, 250, 253, 267, 279, 288, 292
medical care, 30, 59
medical history, 288
medical science, 9
Medicare, vi, viii, 164, 196, 223, 224, 225, 227, 228, 229, 231, 232, 235, 236, 237,

239, 240, 251, 252, 253, 258, 259, 261, 284, 285, 295, 297, 299
medication, 41, 115, 169, 180, 182, 195, 199, 208, 210, 214, 220, 234, 235, 236, 251, 258, 263, 270, 271, 272, 273, 286, 288, 292, 295
medicine, 40, 65, 80, 90, 103, 196, 197, 238, 291
mental health, 229, 235, 239, 242, 276
misuse, x, 128, 135, 164, 167, 168, 176, 177, 178, 179, 180, 187, 191, 192, 193, 194, 196, 199, 224, 252, 278

N

National Survey, 128, 129, 144, 162, 178, 181, 196
natural disaster, 280
negative consequences, 199

O

officials, viii, x, 125, 127, 130, 131, 139, 142, 151, 167, 176, 179, 181, 187, 190, 191, 193, 198, 199
operating costs, ix, 126, 140
operations, 58, 83, 170
opioid epidemic, viii, 125, 127, 225, 227, 296, 298
opioids, vii, viii, x, 33, 53, 54, 55, 125, 127, 128, 144, 145, 146, 147, 170, 172, 176, 177, 178, 179, 180, 182, 183, 184, 185, 186, 187, 188, 189, 190, 191, 192, 193, 194, 195, 196, 197, 198, 199, 224, 233, 237, 240, 242, 243, 250, 252
opportunities, 3, 5, 62, 63, 72, 74, 298
oversight, 11, 28, 37, 74, 130, 171, 182, 227, 249

P

pain, x, 54, 55, 127, 128, 129, 142, 143, 145, 147, 163, 172, 176, 178, 182, 196, 197, 199, 219, 220, 224, 227, 237, 240, 242, 250
pain care, 199
pain management, 143, 237, 240, 242
pathway, 28, 47, 48, 54, 70, 123
permit, 235, 252, 257, 264, 265, 267, 268, 273, 289, 290
pharmacies, viii, 125, 126, 129, 133, 138, 139, 140, 152, 155, 158, 163, 164, 176, 180, 183, 187, 192, 234, 264, 265, 268, 275, 276, 277, 278, 279, 280, 281, 285, 288, 289, 290, 291, 292
pharmacists, viii, 84, 125, 134, 151, 165, 170, 195, 196, 198, 240, 244, 245, 254, 266, 268, 273, 274, 278, 288, 289, 290, 291, 292
physical health, 239
physical properties, 192
physician, viii, 18, 19, 58, 125, 129, 143, 150, 168, 178, 197, 266, 291, 293, 294
policy, vii, x, 59, 75, 123, 137, 138, 162, 167, 168, 201, 229, 230, 233
policymakers, vii, ix, 122, 126, 130, 131, 146, 166, 171
population, vii, x, xi, 45, 46, 47, 103, 106, 114, 115, 128, 143, 145, 162, 176, 179, 180, 181, 187, 188, 195, 201, 202, 203, 204, 206, 207, 208, 209, 210, 213, 220, 224, 279
predictability, 7, 21, 29, 32, 65, 76, 81, 95, 96, 98, 100, 101, 104, 116
prescribers, viii, 87, 125, 126, 131, 132, 139, 143, 144, 146, 147, 148, 149, 162, 164, 167, 198, 199, 235, 237, 240, 275, 276, 277, 279, 280, 281
prescription drug abuse, vii, ix, x, 126, 127, 128, 129, 130, 131, 136, 142, 143, 146,

147, 162, 163, 164, 165, 166, 172, 236, 275, 276, 277, 278, 279, 280, 281, 282, 283
prescription drug monitoring programs (PDMPs), v, vii, viii, 125, 126, 127, 129, 130, 131, 132, 133, 134, 135, 136, 137, 138, 139, 140, 141, 142, 143, 144, 145, 146, 147, 148, 149, 151, 152, 153, 154, 155, 156, 157, 159, 160, 161, 162, 163, 164, 165, 166, 167, 169, 170, 171, 172, 233
prescription drug plan sponsors, vi, viii, 223, 224, 232, 236, 259, 261, 271, 297, 299
prescription drug use patterns, vii, x, 201
Prescription Drug User Fee Act, vii, 2, 4, 12, 64, 78, 97, 98, 99, 105, 116, 117, 120
prescription drugs, viii, x, xi, 62, 125, 129, 130, 131, 137, 144, 145, 147, 153, 154, 163, 172, 187, 201, 202, 203, 204, 205, 206, 207, 208, 209, 213, 214, 215, 216, 217, 218, 219, 220, 233, 271, 278
prescription opioids, v, vii, x, 127, 146, 147, 170, 172, 175, 176, 177, 178, 179, 186, 187, 198
probability, 69, 71, 209, 221, 238
protection, vii, x, 127, 131, 166, 238
proton pump inhibitors, 214, 219
public awareness, 130, 177, 197
public health, viii, 12, 26, 34, 56, 61, 64, 73, 77, 84, 96, 97, 100, 126, 130, 131, 150, 151, 160, 171, 243, 256, 275
public sector, 165
public service, 197, 261

R

race, xi, 201, 204, 206, 207, 209
recommendations, iv, 2, 5, 7, 24, 33, 101, 107, 108, 109, 117, 137, 138, 149, 150, 165, 187, 191, 197, 199, 208, 290
recruiting, 8, 31, 36, 83, 104
regulations, 134, 183, 184, 185, 191, 194, 250, 251, 253, 284, 288, 292
regulatory agencies, 65, 136
regulatory oversight, 14
requirements, 15, 52, 53, 90, 135, 137, 155, 162, 165, 166, 170, 171, 179, 182, 183, 184, 185, 198, 227, 233, 234, 239, 240, 248, 253, 255, 256, 257, 262, 266, 274, 277, 284, 286, 287, 288, 289, 290, 291, 292, 293, 294, 296
researchers, x, 24, 30, 61, 66, 70, 143, 144, 146, 150, 176, 180, 192
resources, 3, 6, 11, 25, 26, 31, 32, 37, 42, 45, 48, 51, 55, 56, 61, 69, 71, 79, 80, 83, 85, 96, 98, 100, 101, 102, 103, 104, 120, 121, 199, 273, 275
response, vii, x, 26, 70, 89, 101, 116, 134, 161, 162, 163, 201, 227, 281, 298
restrictions, 170, 235, 282
retail, 133, 163, 180, 183, 274, 278
revenue, 32, 81, 104, 112, 254
risk, viii, 3, 6, 10, 21, 22, 63, 75, 76, 77, 87, 88, 90, 96, 117, 132, 133, 144, 148, 154, 157, 175, 184, 197, 198, 199, 223, 224, 232, 234, 236, 252, 259, 261, 263, 265, 270, 271, 272, 275, 276, 277, 278, 279, 280, 281, 282, 283, 284, 285, 297, 299
risk assessment, 3, 6, 22, 88
risk management, 21
risks, 10, 75, 79, 88, 93, 102, 103, 163, 182, 184, 240
rules, 34, 35, 116, 138, 264, 265, 283, 284

S

safety, xi, 4, 6, 8, 9, 12, 14, 17, 22, 30, 40, 44, 45, 53, 58, 61, 68, 71, 72, 74, 77, 85, 89, 98, 99, 100, 102, 103, 104, 107, 109, 111, 114, 117, 184, 213, 267, 278, 289

science, 8, 10, 14, 22, 24, 26, 36, 37, 38, 61, 63, 64, 66, 72, 75, 77, 80, 85, 86, 92, 95, 96, 102, 103, 114, 116, 121, 122
scientific method, 102
scientific progress, 63
scientific understanding, 9
Senate, 38, 64, 118, 122, 178, 300
servers, 139
services, iv, 83, 119, 136, 151, 233, 235, 236, 237, 243, 255, 271, 273, 276, 280, 285, 287, 292
sex, xi, 201, 203, 207, 216
side effects, 70, 119, 147
Social Security, vi, viii, 223, 230, 231, 232, 236, 239, 297, 299
Social Security Act, vi, viii, 223, 230, 231, 232, 236, 239, 297, 299
spending, 143, 224, 227, 228, 229, 230, 232, 233, 234, 235, 236, 237, 238, 239, 240, 241, 242, 243, 244, 248, 249, 250, 251, 252, 253, 254, 255
state, viii, ix, x, 3, 5, 62, 74, 78, 125, 126, 127, 128, 130, 131, 132, 133, 134, 135, 136, 137, 138, 139, 140, 141, 143, 147, 150, 151, 154, 155, 156, 157, 158, 159, 161, 162, 163, 164, 168, 169, 170, 171, 179, 180, 183, 185, 195, 230, 233, 234, 244, 255
structure, 3, 6, 32, 43, 50, 56, 81, 104, 112, 262, 288, 293
substance abuse, 132, 145, 150, 170, 171, 227, 229, 239
substance use, 199, 227, 230, 234, 235, 241, 242, 248, 252, 253, 256
substance use disorders, 199, 227, 230, 234, 235, 241, 242, 252, 253, 256

T

target, 32, 56, 57, 58, 70, 84
taxonomy, 28, 71, 93
technical assistance, 139, 152, 161, 237
technological advances, 95
technological change, 30
testing, 34, 36, 67, 68, 69, 71, 164, 180, 193, 209, 239, 243, 291, 297, 299
therapy, 5, 10, 18, 39, 46, 56, 59, 69, 79, 87, 101, 121, 162, 234, 236, 258, 263, 270, 271, 272, 273, 295
training, 90, 91, 135, 152, 165, 184, 198, 242, 244, 253, 292
transparency, 21, 28, 78, 80, 81, 88
treatment, viii, 18, 22, 26, 27, 46, 56, 57, 59, 64, 69, 77, 101, 119, 121, 126, 130, 131, 145, 152, 165, 170, 171, 184, 185, 190, 198, 208, 210, 227, 229, 230, 234, 235, 236, 239, 243, 250, 251, 256, 268, 269, 293, 294
trial, 11, 18, 21, 29, 42, 46, 47, 48, 59, 77, 80, 87, 91, 92, 94, 96, 102, 106, 109, 111, 148

U

uniform, 73, 75, 160, 269, 274, 288, 289, 290, 291, 292
United States, v, xi, 11, 13, 14, 16, 32, 45, 61, 63, 65, 78, 79, 98, 99, 105, 127, 128, 129, 133, 147, 153, 169, 172, 175, 178, 201, 203, 204, 205, 206, 210, 213, 214, 215, 216, 217, 218, 219, 220, 221, 222, 248, 252, 267
user fees, vii, 2, 3, 4, 7, 13, 32, 35, 36, 47, 51, 62, 66, 67, 74, 76, 78, 79, 83, 84, 85, 89, 95, 98, 117, 120, 121, 122, 123

W

witnesses, 4, 6, 8, 9, 11, 60, 96, 116
workforce, 37, 56, 96, 100, 104
workload, 17, 28, 68, 82, 98, 101, 104, 244, 251